CHEMICALISM

I am a Chemaholic

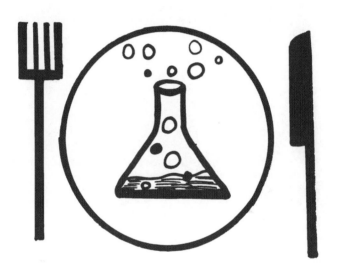

*12 steps to being free
from addiction to artificial chemicals
used in processed food
and drinks*

Simon Kadwill-Kelly

ISBN: 978-0-9933046-0-6

First published in 2016

INDEX

Definition of Chemicalism and Chemaholic 5

Symptoms of a Chemaholic................................6

Who can benefit from this lifestyle change? 8

LBC radio - A chatty explanation 12

Thanks to 19

My Simple Story and Progress...........................22

12 Step Chemaholic Recovery Plan

1 Am I going Crazy 31

2 A leap of faith with courage to take action in a new
direction..63

3 Trust In Nature it really works.....................89

4 List and search for a nutritional SPRING CLEAN!.... 103

5 Announce to yourself and others your new
plan IS underway...................................... 119

6 Exchanging deprivation for ABUNDANCE............... 129

7 Pleasure and stress triggers balanced with humility . 137

8 Look younger by improved natural detoxing 151

9 Enjoy a new level of better health 167

10 Review and adjust 177

11 Resting detox and peaceful balance 189

12 Passing on your enriched lifestyle in order
to attract more well-being 199

Quiz Questions 217

Terms & Quiz Question Answers 226

"WONDEA" Nutritional needs for a
recovering Chemaholic 275

Benefits of Processed Food with artificial chemicals ... 276

Full Dictionary Definitions 2013 278

Research References 282

Books & websites 286

Simon Kadwill-Kelly Medical proof............................ 288

Summary 290

Definition of Chemicalism and Chemaholic

Chemicalism

The subject of artificial Chemically processed food and drink addictive dependence by Human beings and animals.

Chemaholic

A person or animal suffering from Chemicalism. A Chemaholic has:

- Regular compulsive cravings or binge cravings

- Loss of control over the consumption

- Despite negative consequences and withdrawal upon stopping consumption

- Both rewarding and reinforcing

- May not be aware they are a Chemaholic of processed food and drinks made or grown with artificial chemicals.

Full definitions with references are in the appendix

Symptoms of a Chemaholic

1. Frequent strong cravings for processed foods and drinks with artificial chemicals.

2. Bloated full stomach during or after having quickly finished a meal or snack.

3. Repeated attempts to quit some chemaholic foods or set rules to regulate consumption which have always been unsuccessful.

4. Feelings of guilt after eating chemaholic foods then eating the same foods again soon afterwards.

5. Justification by any reason to eat chemaholic foods that are being craved, when known tasty natural food is available.

6. Strong cravings for eating more than originally intended to the point of feeling unwell. Especially after resisting eating chemaholic food for extended periods, when known tasty natural food is available.

7. Justification of choices of food based on low price not high nutrition.

8. Purchase of food based on consumer marketing packaging, advertising or presentation without checking nutritional content.

9. Concealment of consumption or storage of chemaholic foods from others.

10. Inability to control consumption of chemaholic foods, knowing they are causing personal physical harm.

11. A craving for chemaholic foods at times of emotional stress, when a tasty natural food alternative is available.

12. Warnings by a doctor or qualified medical professional that chemaholic eating habits have led to obesity or illness.

These are just twelve common symptoms more are explained in the steps.

This self awareness book offers an easy 12 step practical plan of recovery for chemaholics. This method progressed me from a suffering chemaholic to a happily recovering one.

Who can benefit from this lifestyle change?

When I understood the source of my chemaholic addiction was simply about the desire to feel happy it was a breakthrough. I want to share my positive experiences by keep spreading an easy to follow chemaholic recovery lifestyle. whilst saving money.

Unlike other addictions, eating and drinking are essential for staying alive. The key in these steps is to provide an enjoyable plan. Goals include:

- Maximising natural nutrition
- Allowing for consumption of some low nutrition foods
- Avoiding feelings of deprivation, guilt or fear about enjoying food
- Conveniently available nutrition options

This "How To Overcome" book is for anyone interested in **increasing awareness** of improving their health by reducing regular high consumption of artificial chemicals used in food and drinks.

The audience for this book includes the following:

Anyone interested in weight adjustment long term. Losing weight naturally and effortlessly.

Open minded people ready for a no gimmick method I used to stop suffering from:

- Obesity
- Chronic back ache and occasional acute sciatica
- High cholesterol
- High glucose taking me close to being diabetic type II
- Blood pressure in need of balancing
- Lack of energy
- Regular indigestion

Senior people over 90 years like my mum ready to enjoy food, regain improved health. My mum at 94 years had recovered from:

- Terminal gangrene
- Avoided a leg amputation
- Controlling diabetes type II through nutrition to complete recovery
- High cholesterol
- Leg ulcers

Those who want to save money on food bills, quickly focusing on improved nutrition for proven solutions, and organic-based, ready meals for under £1.00; a free recipe is given in chapter one "I am crazy."

People who are tired of information overload. There is a lot of well written information easily available about how commercially produced fast food meals, processed foods and drinks with artificial chemicals can have a negative effect on a person's well-being. **That being accepted as true**, this book avoids dwelling on the published negative side effects and looks at quick solutions through simple steps.

Busy people who need a book that is written to be read and with solutions that can be put into action quickly.

Those interested or totally ready for a down-to-earth, low cost solution for improved health with no requirement for special equipment or athletic exercise.

People who may wish to look years younger; this goal provides a simple starting point.

The book also touches upon cancer and how nutrition has been used as a cure, but this book can make no health claims for legal reasons. There are many excellent testimonial books by people who have written about possible ways of curing some types of cancer, which fits in with the simple approach in my book about getting started with basics of a personalised lifestyle change.

Carers and parents who have a passion to improve people's lives with high nutrition.

Those who need a plan of detoxing generally, including through improved, cleansing sleep.

LBC Radio - A chatty explanation

24th June 2015 Transcription

Nick Abbott Radio Presenter Chatting with Simon Kadwill-Kelly about Chemicalism and Chemaholics

Nick: Simon.

Simon: Hello, good morning.

Simon: I was very interested to hear that you're talking about chemicals, in the food, the way it gets in there, and how it gets incorporated into the drugs that I'm told cure us all. And I feel very lucky because, just over two years ago, I had took some advice from a lady about eating natural products, and it's just changed my life completely, and for the better.

Nick: What products are you talking about?

Simon: I used to eat and drink a lot of products with chemicals in them. I thought they were quite good for me, because I'd always go for things with healthy-looking labels, but I realised that the microwave food I used to eat had a whole load of things in it and I just didn't read the small print.

Nick: Yeah. So you stopped eating microwave food, essentially meals that had been pre-prepared and you just heat up, right? What are you eating now?

Simon: Well, still microwave meals, but I make them myself with organic vegetables.

Nick: So the way in which you cook them hasn't changed, it's just that you're cooking from scratch?

Simon: Correct.

Nick: Right. Well, that has to be the way. It used to be, until relatively recently, that every meal was made from scratch because we didn't have convenience foods.

Simon: I admit, when I get hungry, I just have to eat. And I just need to grab food and eat it, and that has been my downfall in the past, having a big appetite.

Nick: Snacking.

Simon: Well, I do that now, but I'm three-and-a-half stone lighter. I eat more than I used to. I'm not fearful of eating food now. I just figure that if you eat about 80% of the good stuff, you can eat other stuff, and it doesn't really impact on you too much.

Nick: You know, every now and again, somebody will come up with a new diet, and the most recent one is a form of starving yourself. They had the five-two thing, where you would eat almost nothing at all for two days, and then stuff cake in your face for five, and now they're saying, "No, that's not right, you shouldn't be doing that. You should be eating more, rather than starving yourself for two days, you should be eating more food, but for longer." No, wait a minute, I'll see if I've got this right.

Simon: There is a bit of a merry-go-round with all the different options, and I think that's all just part of it. I came to the conclusion that it was about time to invent a word to try to encompass this. So I came up with a new word.

Nick: Well, release it to the world, Simon. Lay it on us. What's that word?

Simon: Chemicalism. I've defined it as the subject of being addicted to chemical food. I would call myself a "chemaholic." Crazy as it may sound, I certainly was full-on with it. I would say now that I am only just mildly addicted.

Nick: You're a recovering "chemaholic," right?

Simon: Yeah. And I keep surprising myself. I went out the other day, and I had a couple of meals at a restaurant, and it just kicked off. I just found I was consuming. I just had a nice meal at lunchtime, Chinese, had Italian in the evening, and before I knew it, I was just ravenous for anything that had lots of sugar and chemicals.

Nick: Well, of course the Chinese meal would be chock-full of MSG, no?

Simon: Well, whatever it's full of, and I wouldn't really like to know, to be honest, I definitely enjoyed it. And I think enjoying food is really important.

Nick: You'll probably enjoy it more if you don't know what's in it. Yeah, you're probably right about that.

Simon: Definitely. So, I think that the key to it all is taking just a few extra moments to check where it comes from.

Nick: And, as you say, to cook from scratch. Because it's not that hard. I mean Jamie blooming Oliver, there's barely a moment of the day where he's not on TV in some form or other, showing you how to cook from scratch in three seconds or less.

Simon: I think the problem is that, a lot of the cooking programmes look great, but when it comes down to it, I feel there's a lot of people like me who just get hungry and who will eat straight away because they have a busy lives. The way I've gotten around it is, about every couple of weeks, I make about 20 or 30 meals, then freeze them all...

Nick: That's what I was going to say, yeah...

Simon: ...and spread them out.

Nick: Yeah, exactly right.

Simon: A friend of mine, a very big guy, said, "I love the idea, but it's too expensive to eat organic." Because he's a computer person, I made him a spreadsheet for one of my boil up and cook meals, and it worked out at 84 pence for a 450 millilitre container of food, which is a meal for me. And that was buying it from a well-known, big store that sells organic stuff and vegetables at retail prices.

Nick: 82p?

Simon: 84p. Actually, I told him that was 99p per meal. He said, "That's not true." I said, "You're right, it's 84p."

Nick: Well, it's a good idea to cook 20 meals at a time, just as long as you don't eat all 20 as soon as you've cooked them! So you bag them up and you put them in the freezer?

Simon: It's actually very interesting that you say that because you get two types of chefs, thin ones and ones that are big. Often chefs, after doing all the cooking, don't actually feel that hungry. I've found I do a whole load of cooking for about an hour and half, or may be two hours.

Nick: And then that's the last thing you want to eat! Yeah, I understand that.

Simon: Yeah.

Nick: All right, thanks a lot, Simon. You know, it's not so weird that he would be addicted to food, because the food manufacturers do have men in white coats in laboratories, whose job it is to come up with the perfect combination of fats and salts and sugars and so on, which makes it impossible to stop eating their products. Have you ever opened a bag of something and thought, "Mmm, so yummy?" Before you opened the bag, you were convinced that you were just going to have a couple of whatever it might be, and then re-seal the bag and put it in the cupboard.

And you found how difficult it is to do that? Well, it's not a coincidence. They have deliberately engineered food to make it impossible to stop eating. It's addictive by design. One of the things that I've got a bee in my bonnet about is that the human race is being poisoned. As I said, we've changed shape. And that is undeniable. Look around, the high street did not look like this 20 years ago.

People haven't really changed their lifestyles that much. The explosion in gyms has happened relatively recently. If you went to a gym in the 1970s, it would have been a relatively unusual thing to do, and the gym would probably have been full of Arnold Schwarzenegger body builder types. They weren't full of people from the office just having a class for half an hour.

Such a thing (the new types of gyms) didn't really exist. They were pretty awful places full of clanging dumbbells and machinery. These days, there's barely a main street in the country that doesn't have one or two gyms on it. People are exercising more than they used to do.

Radio FM 97.3 MHz - London - www.lbc.co.uk

Thanks To

Dad

Who always encouraged me to be creative and carry on with determination without fear of failure. His saying to me: *"He who dares, slims."*

Mum

For everything that I could wish of a good mum. Plus having an open mind at 93 yrs young to adopt in 2013 a life saving natural nutrition lifestyle. My mum astounded medical professionals by avoiding a leg amputation from terminal gangrene which was cured naturally in 2014. Peeling the vegetables for home made recipes and organic microwave meals.

Mr A.S. Jibawi (Vascular consultant & Surgeon)

Who believed and supported my mum's determination to have better health.

Liz Cappetta Naturopathic Nutritional Therapist

For all the excellent nutrition advice given to my mum about new ways to enjoy food and understand natural healing.

Elsa Wakeling International simultaneous interpreter

Introducing me to "Normal Food" over a period

of weeks based on Elsa's Lifetime of Naturopathy Lifestyle with a modern day twist. This led to my easy weight loss of 22 kilos over six months in 2013. Saying goodbye to high cholesterol, high blood pressure, tinnitus, borderline diabetic type II and becoming generally well with more energy to enjoy a healthier Lifestyle.

Nick Wood, BSc, PhD, PGCLTHE, FHEA, GPhC, MPSI, MRSC

Who simply pointed me to an unscientific 30 day humorous experiment documented in Morgan Spurlock's film "Supersize Me" to help me explain better Chemicalism & Chemaholics to everyday people like me who enjoy the convenience of tasty foods.

Graham Richards

Who believed people should have the best information to make informed decisions about what is right for them and to shout out the truth with passion when it can change people's lives for the better.

Yinka Udueni

The best Pharmacist my mum, dad and I have ever met who takes time to explain how medicines work and reviewed my mum's medicine every few months whilst my mum decreased the tablet prescriptions.

Dr Nick Merrifield, General Practitioner Doctor

Who gave me a prescription for a three month NHS Gym course to lose weight and get fit.

Magdalena Pryce, MA - Personal Trainer www.mprycetraining.com

Exercise Referral Instructor in Public Health (NHS). For explaining that 20% of exercise and 80% of high nutritional food is responsible for weight loss. Motivating me to better fitness whilst I was recovering from a major shoulder operation.

Shirley Rhodes International healer

Who quietly goes about healing people and animals through her natural Elixir for life. Plus her quotes in step 11 which give a clearer meaning to an unscientific subject

Nick Abbot, LBC Radio (London)

On a Live LBC Radio conversation 24th June 2015 Nick gave me the chance to launch to the world two new words "Chemicalism" and "Chemaholic," offering listeners a clear meaning to the subject of "Addiction to artificial chemical food & drinks" through these new words.

My Simple Story and Progress

Obese at age 52, working fulltime in IT Support, being a carer, plus studying to increase my Microsoft IT qualifications gave me a busy life. I discovered in under six months during 2013 a convenient new Lifestyle combining both high and low nutrition foods. This new Lifestyle helped me lose 22 kilos in six months effortlessly, weight which I believe is gone long term. I have said goodbye to many unwanted health conditions, including high cholesterol, close to being diabetic type II, lack of energy. This is without deprivation of my favourite tastes or places to enjoy eating.

Since my mid-twenties, I have experienced typical physical side effects as a chemaholic with blood tests showing high cholesterol and sugar levels.

This lead to my search through a merry go round of many trendy pills, diets and exercises for a solution to reduce weight and have deeper sleep and extra energy.

The biggest impact on my hard working life has been years of lower back and sciatic acute pain, making me disabled and unable to walk at two periods in my life. Classed by the State as officially disabled in my 30's and unable to work, I set about finding a solution without surgery, a solution which I thankfully found. Once cured,

I returned to fulltime work, got a motorbike, started sailing and have never looked back!

Private and NHS(National Health Service – UK) Orthopaedic Consultants took MRI Scans of my lower back, showing, in their opinion, degenerated discs that would stop me from being able to walk again properly until I received a major spine operation. I said No! The chances of a successful spine surgery with published high success rates taking away the disabling pain were attractive. However, I had not been able to find anyone post spine operation with a completely successful result, so with the fear of possibly being wheel chair bound, my search continued for a natural solution which came about mainly through high nutrition food. This was my first life changing experience that simple homemade meals were able to heal.

I believe over consumption of artificial chemicals in my nutrition largely contributed to inflammation in my lower spine, causing acute pain because after a few days of detoxing by consuming only raw vegetable soup, juicing and purified water, the pain always subsides. Most people relate to this in terms of over consumption of alcohol followed by quick fix detoxing by drinking extra water and maybe some pills to speed up uncomfortable recovery. I gave up alcohol and smoking in 2000 which gave me an insight into addictive behaviour.

The cocktail of artificial chemicals in food plus pills to counter the side effects of them had made me into a human laboratory, overloaded with trying to process and filter the laboratory chemicals.

Up to 2012, my knowledge about nutrition and exercise followed the popular main stream beliefs offered by helpful UK Government information. Food sellers of all kinds also provided me with information on their packaging about ingredients often complemented with a healthy looking message. I was getting more overweight, often hungry, fearful of eating, drinking lots of water, eating vegetables each day. I started to believe my body was failing and visited my local doctor for answers, expecting a prescription of tablets to fix some part of my body, but I had a surprise when given something completely different !

My doctor Nick Merrifield gave me an NHS prescription for a three month gym membership called a " Get Active Exercise Referral Programme."

At the first gym induction session, Magdalena the instructor explained that due to my bandaged shoulder recovering from a recent major operation. I was not allowed to exercise fully in the gym, so instead we spent the first few sessions mainly discussing nutrition which Magdalena convinced me was more important than exercising when it comes to having a healthy lifestyle and weight loss.

Then I met a good friend Elsa who opened my mind to a much easier way of living with more energy, faster thinking, better immunity, balanced weight, and a younger outlook. She challenged my old beliefs, explaining *I was crazy* eating so much artificial chemically processed nutrition, and I could benefit from eating "Normal Food" instead.

During 2013 gradually learning about "Normal Foods" from Elsa, I switched to eating mainly organic nutrition plus gluten free for the biscuits, cakes and chocolates. Weight started to fall off effortlessly after six weeks whilst energy levels increased.

Regular blood tests every few weeks showed cholesterol and glucose were consistently dropping down. Weight decreased by 22 kilos (nearly 3 stone 7lbs) over six months, which Dr Merrifield was pleased to report on my medical records.

Late 2013 on vacation in Malta, my addictive desire for artificial chemical food took off with the tasty artificial chemical style 3* hotel food causing weight gains at the rate of 3 kilos per week. One day I swam two hours in the sea nonstop across Mellieha Bay. Then walked back three hours from the town St. Julian's to my hotel the same evening expecting to shed some weight. This was the most exercise I had enjoyed for years. Instead, I continued to gain weight and enjoy an increasing amount of hotel food that just was not filling me up like the home made organic meals I had become used to.

Still on vacation with an extra big unexpected appetite for breakfast. I had a moment of inspiration hit me in a flash! In just a week I had reignited my strong addiction to artificial chemical food based on my old values. I am a Chemaholic !

This moment of sudden honest self realisation made complete sense to me that *Chemicalism creates* Chemaholics. Physical and mental addiction to artificial chemical processed nutrition was the truth I had long searched for. Knowing there were many proven twelve step addiction recovery programs. I realised a 12 step recovery plan from artificial chemical addiction was possible to apply into my life to enjoy a healthier lifestyle.

I am tremendously grateful to have enjoyably changed to a healthier lifestyle having lost a lot of weight long term, enjoying more energy, and seeing my mum's health improve after being diagnosed with terminal gangrene back in 2012.

It is my privilege to share this experience so far during my lifetime of learning.

Many diet and exercise advertisements are geared to successful short term weight loss involving some hardship and or deprivation of tasty foods and drinks. The facts are these diets are only successful over a few weeks or months. This is because of the dieters' craving for the foods and habits they had become used to for many years based on their unhelpful nutrition knowledge.

On returning to the previous low nutrition diet, the failed dieter feels comforted, rewarded with their old habits usually with a sense of it was their fault because they did not have enough will power. This merry go round circus ride of weight loss diet cycles is repeated with many diet types; often with the same results. This keeps the growing multibillion-pound diet and healthcare industry very profitable whilst governments doing their best to cope with a growing number of patients; this provides many jobs. My experience of trying lots of weight loss diets and exercise programs over many years was very disheartening.

The shortcut I discovered for losing weight was to stop trying out different weight loss options. Instead, I changed my attitude towards nutrition, gradually incorporating new enjoyable eating habits. The results took more than the typical

30 day diets. However, the benefits of swapping to mainly natural foods started around six weeks later. I invested extra thoughtfulness into discovering high nutrition foods whilst changing my habits.

This 12 step program is a lifestyle change which very importantly includes the tasty foods you enjoy, exercise is secondary to an improved well being. In my case lost me 22 kilos in six months during 2013. I did not believe the lifestyle change would work as I had failed at so many weight loss diets. Every few weeks I had a doctors check up with blood samples. I no longer wanted to be borderline diabetic type II, officially obese, with high blood pressure and high cholesterol. I needed facts from the blood tests regularly to prove my new attitude towards nutrition confirmed I was a happily recovering chemaholic.

Saving money I had not anticipated would be one of the many benefits as all I wanted to do was lose weight and avoid being diabetic. My outgoings unexpectedly reduced firstly with home cooking by making batches of tasty organic ready meals every week or two which I froze. This cut down my food bill when I had expected to be spending more.

When I was very obese, my trips to the doctors, hospital consultants, chemists and health stores, buying supplements and prescriptions, was normal every few days. It felt so strange as these tasks tailed off after about eight weeks later, giving me more free time to enjoy. I used to be paid on a contract day rate. I noticed my new better health meant less illness and put more cash in my pocket within a few weeks; which just made me more enthusiastic. Also, I had been used to suffering from side effects from the pain killer drugs I no longer required for physical pains. This meant I no longer needed other medicines or purchase natural remedies to counteract the side effects.

Medical Disclaimer

All content in this book are for information purposes only. The Content is not intended to be a substitute for professional medical advice, diagnosis, or treatment. Always seek the advice of your physician or other qualified health provider with any questions you may have regarding a medical condition. Never disregard professional medical advice or delay in seeking it because of something you have read in this book. There is no representation, no responsibility, liability or warranties, express or implied, about the completeness, accuracy, reliability, suitability or availability with respect to the information, products, services in this book. Before starting any diet, you should speak to your doctor. This information is not intended to be patient education, does not create any patient-physician relationship, and should not be used as a substitute for professional diagnosis, tests and treatment.

STEP 1

"Am I going Crazy ?"

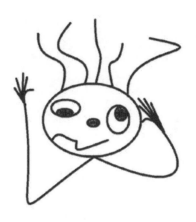

"Insanity is doing the same thing over and over again and expecting a different result."

Albert Einstein

"It's better to face madness with a plan than to sit still and let it take you in pieces."

Josh Malerman, Bird Box

"All living things contain a measure of madness that moves them in strange, sometimes inexplicable ways."

Yann Martel, Life of Pi

"There nearly always is a method in madness."

G.K. Chesterton

To get a healthier lifestyle, I first had to honesty admit to myself

"I am a Chemaholic"

then let the truth set me free! I wanted to be free from the mental and physical addiction of artificial chemical foods.

Sick and tired of being Sick and Tired made me decide on taking a leap of faith with changing my attitude towards nutrition, following new beliefs from which other people had already benefited to get a healthy lifestyle.

Swapping to a mix of high and low nutrition foods for a convenient healthier new lifestyle long term has made sense because sometimes circumstances dictate what food options are available, such as on holiday.

Every day as far as I remember up to 2012, I was mainly consuming artificial chemically processed food and drink, expecting to become healthier and slimmer. My strong beliefs and values justified defensively my knowledge, which kept me stuck in a repetitive self-destructive merry go round loop of increasing obesity. This was crazy. I was crazy. Only by accepting I am a Chemaholic would enable change to a new happier lifestyle.

Admitting honestly, I am a chemaholic unable to go from day to day without a chemical food fix signified a turning point. I started changing habits gradually each week for one month, preparing for what I understood at the time as a detox. Allowing a month on STEP ONE to get ready for STEP TWO was good timing. I recommend a month of mental preparation coupled with developing new habits to increase the chances of reaching STEP TWO.

If you are wondering if you are a Chemaholic, be your own best judge by :

- Write on a sheet of paper, your blood test results, study for just 10 minutes

- BMI (weight & height) calculation, check what is considered average

- Make a detailed list of EVERY medicine stocked or used to provide facts

- List any medical complaints, highlight ones associated with obesity

- Symptoms of a Chemaholic, how many are you suffering from

Then armed with the facts truthfully ask yourself with an open mind, then your doctor. Would a change in nutrition consumption with less artificial chemicals

plus an increase of natural foods be likely to reduce any suffering?

My new lifestyle fortunately was motivated by my friend Elsa; I was impressed with her many years of younger looks due to high nutritional eating with an energetic lifestyle that she adopted many years ago. Elsa had just passed a physical fitness test in 2013 to become a fitness instructor with a well-known chain of Leisure Centres so this proved to me she would be an excellent mentor.

In brief, the main points of step one:

Taking personal responsibility. It was up to me to know and assess what I consume not relying upon packaging, government information, an authority, any business or personal recommendation but by gaining better knowledge about nutrition, better choices for nutrition have come about.

Knowing the real source of the food and drink. Has it been processed, grown with artificial chemicals? If Fish and animals - what were they being fed with?

Buying food based on price not nutrition. Bargains, special offers, cheap value for money food and drinks must be of less importance than nutritional value. Organic products with no artificial chemicals are more valuable than price or perceived quality due to advertising.

Avoiding the purchase of more than required, saving money. Storing fresh vegetables decreases nutrition each day of storage unless frozen to lock in nutrition. Avoid eating foods just to comply with out of date deadlines. No longer be afraid to throw away food which is low nutrition or not fresh because it has a financial value or to please another person. Please your own health first.

Eating large meals when feeling full to avoid wasting food or pleasing somebody is no longer valuable. Stopping eating when feeling full enough is now very valuable for improved digestion.

Being aware of advertising & healthy looking packaging with attractive messages for artificial chemical food and drink. My own increased awareness has made me feel more responsible to question the validity of these enticing words, not to buy with only my eyes. Here are some examples of attractive adverting messages for some artificial chemical foods with low nutrition:

- Freshly made

- Free range

- Hand Made

- Homemade

- Healthy

- No added Salt or Reduced Salt

- Fat free or Reduced Fat

- Contains only artificial sweeteners or reduced sugar

- Reduced Calorie - Low calorie

- Made in or produced in a trusty sounding place or country

- Endorsed by a celebrity, cartoon character, healthy looking image

- Pasteurised

- Style, colour, quality or function of packaging

- Added vitamins and minerals
- High in Fibre

There are many attractive ways products are promoted as being healthy. The World Health Organisation recognises this and introduced advertising guidelines for products being marketed to children.

(Natural Organic foods tend to promote just that main label of being organic without any gimmicky advertising message to persuade buyers it is maybe healthier)

The place where food is sold has a big impact on decision making. For example salad products sold in a small shop, a big superstore, an expensive hotel restaurant, a brand name fast food take away or a country farm shop may all suggest a healthy way of shopping but how can you tell? Each step explains more.

Measure your starting point & review in six weeks to confirm your level of success

Step one is about being sure if you have decided you are a Chemaholic through your open minded examination of the facts. Checking your attitude and awareness towards nutrition based partly on facts including blood tests.

Book a health check with a doctor or hospital for a full blood test; confirm blood pressure, weight and anything else you feel is important. See the results and meet a doctor, nurse or health professional to discuss the results in detail: especially for:

- Cholesterol
- Blood Sugar – glucose
- Liver Function
- Kidney Function
- Blood pressure
- Weight
- BMI

Be sure what the actual results are, just get the facts; write them down in your diary. You may be able to get the results in writing if you ask. Do not accept vague opinions such as:

- Nothing to worry about
- The results are about average for your age
- It looks like you need to do some exercise
- Too much alcohol may be causing a poor result
- You may need some medication to improve the results

Exercise in some way, walk for 10 minutes; make a note of how far you got and make a note on a scale of 1 – 10 how tired you felt. Do an exercise you are able to easily re measure. After six weeks, repeat to check for improvement.

After six weeks of lifestyle changes, redo the blood tests to check for improvement.

Ask advice from a qualified personal trainer about doing a specific type of fitness tests or body check, e.g. waist measurement, waist to hip ratio, or body composition and re measure six weeks later to recognise improvement.

A naturopathic doctor or qualified Nutritional Therapist is a good person to seek an opinion about natural remedies and lifestyle changes. Especially when the blood tests or existing medical condition/s strongly suggest Chemicalism has a controlling impact over your life. Show the blood test results to the medical or fitness professional to give them the facts to base good advice upon.

Most people believe any addiction just requires a single person's strong willpower to overcome it. This attitude is highly unlikely to succeed long term. The root cause of addictions is a desire for a mood change. Successful ongoing recovery is about having a new attitude, allowing change to a happier healthy lifestyle.

Check your answers about being a chemaholic in step 10 and see how your scores compare when you have started receiving the benefits of your new lifestyle during the next few weeks.

Starting The Solution

Cutting down consuming pesticides and artificial chemical where possible.

Making lifestyle changes are best done gradually so mind and body accept the adjustment. This book is a quick introduction to the steps in order to bring about a noticeable change in attitude without having to become an expert on nutrition.

Water. It is essential to cut out 99% of microbiological contaminants when consuming water as the body is made up of between 50 -75 % water. Undoubtedly, water is our most important ingredient after oxygen. Humans can stay alive for many weeks without food but not water.

Drink when thirsty so as to not overwork the body organs. Non purified tap water (with pesticides to kill weeds and bacteria) or water from plastic bottles have be proven to contain many containments that require removing before drinking so the body is able to operate in a natural way.

Water entering the body must be within a healthy PH level not over acidic or alkaline.

Many processed foods with artificial chemicals stimulate thirst; one train of thought is that high salt content causes this. With more natural food and drinks introduced, the body becomes more reliably tuned, which is highly likely to reduce thirst.

Cook – boil or better still steam vegetables with purified water 99 +% free of contaminants especially when curing illnesses or seeking weight loss.

To get 99+% purified water, the water source has to be filtered through filters which state they remove 99+% of contaminants. As this saves money with no longer needing to buy bottled water, this is a good investment. There are handheld bottles typically costing £25.00, but again be sure the filters take out 99% of impurities. These can be purchased online and most good camping shops selling survival equipment. There are many nicely packaged water filter products on offer which may provide some improvement but with water you need to treat yourself to the best; to function at your best.

It is possible to put natural trace minerals back into the purified water but at step one the main objective is keep it simple by maximising the reduction of contaminants in drinking and cooking water.

For convenience I have opted for a standalone unit which purifies 10 litres at a time plus a hand held bottle which I keep in the car as well as take on holidays. There filters that can be plumbed in and last a year before the filter requires changing. Check the filter in detail to be sure it takes out 99% of contaminants as there are many which do not.

Buying higher nutrition organic meat and vegetables (unless a vegan or religious reasons) and using them all up almost immediately with no wastage provides maximum nutrition. At first doing so seemed strange, and now I find this normal.

Buying organic and gluten free foods without attention to price was the first biggest hurdle to breaking my addition. I did not realise the supermarkets I had used for many years also had a gluten free section. Natural food from my experience is more filling so after a while I was spending less on food. Buy on nutrition value not monetary value otherwise you will be poor in health.

Throwing away all the frozen/refrigerated/ tinned foods that were laced with artificial chemicals were not an option that my strong value of using up the cost of food would allow. Instead, I used it all up mainly in the first month while studying and listing the chemicals that were being put into my food. I was searching for the evidence to understand artificial chemical additives. Making a gradual adjustment to my new lifestyle allowed my body to adjust, withdraw safely, smoothly. This subject is covered in Step four.

Alcohol is a strong toxin which puts strain on your liver as it filters blood. Drinking Purified water with organic lemon each day is one option to help clean up the liver a little or just once after sleeping to start the day. With life threatening health conditions that require a person to detox in hospital, alcohol is taken out of the menu. Keeping consumption lower maybe easier as your health improves because of a better feeling of well being. To reduce alcohol intake it can be mixed with other non toxic liquids for example ancient Romans used to mix wine with water. Drinking alcohol after eating a meal may reduce the desire to consume as much alcohol and food.

Making my own tasty organic ready meals in batches is easy every two weeks. I use organic vegetables and chicken seasoned with many different flavours. Washed and boiled (steamed in a cooker locks in nutrition) in purified water. The cost (2014) per 450 ml vegetable meal is

84p, with organic chicken £1.23. It saves me money and food preparation time when I grab a meal from the freezer. Having organic fast food instant meals within minutes has kept me on track with long term weight loss and reduced cholesterol levels to normal.

Hunger timing – be ready

Knowing your times of the day when hunger is likely to be high making you more susceptible to eating the first easy options available within a few minutes makes planning ahead easier. I usually have organic apples, nuts and a hand held purifying water bottle in my car or travel bag ready for a snack whilst on the go. This also saves money and time.

Exercise

Exercise comes down to personal motivation which is largely stimulated by the amount of physical energy the body feels the need to use up. Consuming more natural food and drinks produces increased natural energy. Whatever exercise that can be enjoyed is all part of a happy lifestyle. Exercise produces natural chemicals in the brain, dopamine, giving a sense of happy well-being. This increase of more physical energy in most people leads to a more natural weight. The body wants to burn off the natural food energy faster.

The extra energy from consuming more natural food made me feel mentally younger so I started doing many things I used to enjoy 20 years ago. Listening to dance music. Wearing different clothes, shoes. Become more confident with changing around lifestyle options, starting with small things, attract more confidence to take on bigger challenges.

Magda my "Get Active" personal trainer on prescription emphasised daily physical activities are important. They also help me moderately challenge myself, improving my cardiovascular system; strengthening both muscle and bone structure. It is not necessary to visit the gym every day. It is best to just keep moving as much as possible by doing whatever exercise, however moderate, challenging or is most enjoyable. This all works towards improvements for a healthier lifestyle.

There is a great emphasis in many well put together weight loss programs to highly exercise often at a gym or with a sport. This may fit in well with some people's lifestyles. The main thing is to eat more natural foods, which produces natural energy, stimulating a desire to enjoy extra movement.

Eating with our eyes

I keep practicing this awareness everyday by being mindful of eating one mouthful of food at a time. Chewing double the amount of times to improve natural digestion in the mouth increases flavour. I aim to keep my hands off the knife, fork, spoon, chop sticks or food until I have fully eaten each mouthful. This sounds simple, but I have found it takes a lot of ongoing practice to enjoy eating one mouthful at a time to avoid gulping down swallowing undigested, not chewed food. (More about this in the other steps.)

The stomach relies upon the teeth plus many of the mouth's natural chemical enzymes to break down food ready for high easy nutritional absorption. Avoid consuming food quickly, gulped down too fast. The natural 20 minute time delay before the brain is told by the stomach chemicals how full it is gets by- passed. The feeling full process after the initial 15 - 20 minutes continues for about another 10 -30 minutes then slowly decreases over the next two – five hours to build up a natural appetite again.

Benefits of digesting food in the mouth include tasting more flavour, enjoying a longer eating time with less food, avoiding indigestion and or bloating. With soups and homemade meals, I normally use a small spoon to eat, keeping me mindful of digesting better with maximum flavour.

Supplements

We live in a pill popping society, and there are times when, short term, this is useful and or convenient.

These supplements from my local health shop I used since 2012 to aid my body to get kick started with higher nutrition each day, increasing energy. (I am not recommending anyone takes pills but having an awareness of them may be helpful).

Q10 Coenzyme

Coenzyme Q10 is made naturally by the human body, helping cells to produce energy acting as an antioxidant, which improves immunity. I have found after 30 days my energy levels are noticeably increased.

The Nobel Prize in Chemistry 1978 was awarded to Peter Mitchell "for his contribution to the understanding of biological energy transfer through the formulation of the chemiosmotic theory". www.nobelprize.org

This supplement is available in many different qualities.

Probiotics

These supplements are live bacteria and yeasts offered as having different health benefits for several medical conditions, both preventative and treating. They are often consumed in real natural yoghurts or taken as food supplements. Probiotics sometimes described as "good" or "friendly" bacteria for the gut. They can be homemade. Antibiotics are useful in medicine to kill unwanted bacteria. Most prescribed antibiotics also kill the good essential bacteria used to absorb nutrition at the same time. Therefore, having some kind of probiotic after a course of antibiotics assists in generating good bacteria to aid a faster healthy recovery.

Amino Acids

Humans produce some amino acids with the others coming from food. It is essential to obtain enough amino acids every day in food to have a properly functioning body. This is a big subject. The main point is that a low nutrition chemaholic diet is deficient in amino acids. Considering a multi amino acid supplement maybe the way to help kick start a body into working better due to a lack of these essential acids or simply coping with periods of low nutrition.

Chemically synthesized vitamin supplements

Food vitamin supplements purchased in packets, bottles, powders made in a laboratory are not part of a natural food diet. The manufactured chemical supplements only show similar qualities. When the vitamins are live within the real food, they have their maximum valuable natural interaction with live starches, proteins and fats.

Modern day lifestyles with low nutrition foods means the variety of marketed supplements thrive on being a convenient way of aiming to improve personal nutrition. In some lifestyles or medical situations, it may be the only way to get essential vitamins. They play a very valuable role in modern day scientific medicine.

My understanding is the liquid isotonic vitamin supplements and digestive enzymes supplements are much better as a higher amount of nutrition is absorbed faster.

Common reasons people use to justify being a chemaholic with some suggested ways to overcome them with attitude and action

"When it is obvious that the goals cannot be reached don't adjust the goals adjust the action steps."

Confucius, Chinese Philosopher

Courage to start making a change today with any useful action towards your goals, however small, is MORE valuable than gathering information.

• I think they are too expensive	Please see the free recipe in the chapter 84p per 450 ml meal. Make 10 meals to freeze, work out the cost per meal. You are taking out the packaging and advertising costs which normally make natural food much cheaper.

• I have no or little time to prepare meals	Preparing batches of 20 – 40 meals then lock in the nutrition through freezing saves times later each day with instant meal preparation There are ready made organic options if money is not an obstacle.
• I have no storage space	Clearing some space in the freezer for organic meals to replace the artificial chemical food is an option. Tinned Organic options.
• I have no money until state Benefit /pension is available to spend	Prepare to save money with homemade organic cooking, getting the shopping list, pots to cook & containers to store frozen meals already in advance of payday. Start growing vegetables or getting involved with a community allotment.
• I need convenience	Make or buy organic ready meals, deserts and snacks.

• I know that natural food goes off quicker	Eat or cook & freeze organic meals. Eat the natural food soon after purchase.
• I have a family or partner	Enlist the support of family members who want better health to organise convenient menu options to save time, producing extra leisure time. Provide babies, young and elderly family members with high nutrition foods to maximise immunity. Make them the reason not the excuse. When there is no support wait until step five to announce your lifestyle change.

• I need to know how	One versatile foundation recipe is included in this first chapter which involves boiling or steaming vegetables before adding a range of favourite flavours. There is a YouTube video to show an example; see recipe. There are organic readymade food options, for example tinned soup.
• I live with elderly persons or am an elderly person with special food requirements	Food for elderly people needs to be what the person wants to enjoy and able to consume; for example, it may require being extra soft or of different flavours.

• I think organic food is the same as normal food but a higher price	UK & USA laws allow food providers to mark their products with proof it is organic, which is a carefully licensed checked process. The standards from country to country do vary. Artificial chemical additives are shown on packaging normally with number references. E numbers. (excluding pesticides and livestock farming foods additives)
• I do not understand "gluten free"	Free of gluten but usually free of many artificial chemicals provides a more natural product. Bread, Cakes, biscuits, bread can be gluten free.
• I cannot leave home though disability or work	Home delivery by supermarkets and specialist organic food delivery businesses.

• I think a new gadget is responsible for personal high nutrition and has to be used.	Gadgets are helpful; often a fun gimmick such as an electric powered non-essential juicer is a convenient aid for saving time. Gadgets do not need to be held responsible or relied upon for lifetime natural nutrition food preparation.
• I drink bottled water to avoid chemicals	Bottled water has different qualities of purity which range from tap water quality to spring water from the source. Plastic containers interact with the contents especially when warmed up. Read the bottle and check the source. Glass bottles are the best for storing purified water.

• I use tap water for cooking	Organic food is best not washed with tap water to keep chemicals such as weed killer from entering into the food preparation. Boiling the water containing pesticides, anti-bacterial chemicals, traces of lead, fluoride, chlorine does not guarantee these chemicals, contaminants will be removed. Water purification products are able to remove up to 99% of contaminants.
• I am too old to start	Get blood tests, ask doctors' opinions and about treatment Prescriptions & treatments: ask like a child Why? Why? Why? Consult with a professional Naturopath or qualified Naturopathic Doctor for natural remedies and lifestyle improvements.

• I can't afford to use or join a gym or fitness class for exercise	Exercise is free. It is helpful in many cases to join in with others for motivation or choose a nice environment, but always remember exercise can be done anywhere for free.
• I am a people pleaser	Making choices or actions might be based on what people think, want or expect from you. By pleasing one person, you may naturally disappoints another. Look after your own needs first. Love yourself for increased self esteem reinforced with getting physically healthier.

• I am not good enough to deserve high nutrition foods	The low self esteem driving this opinion may be overcome with many positive therapies. To achieve physical results from a new high nutrition lifestyle will aid raising self esteem, improving the chemical function of the mind.
• Personal Reasons • Family Reasons • Any reason that justifies consuming low nutrition	Have faith these can be overcome with some action to get started.
• Analysis Is Paralysis	Analysing in great detail before starting a natural food lifestyle change is disabling. Being a perfectionist may be overcome by starting now.

Organic Ready Meals for under £1.00 with ten different flavours

"Enjoy the taste of your healthy ready meals with high nutrition at a low price "

Enjoy 5 star food @ 2 star prices

This is one of my favourite "Foundation Recipes"

Heating up from frozen in around six minutes

Then add extra flavour and change consistency depending on what I want

ORGANIC LABELLED	Retail Price per pack UK£	Grams
Carrot	1.00	700
Broccoli	1.25	300
Leak	1.00	500
Potatoes	2.00	2 KG
Kale	1.50	200
Baked Bean	0.60	420(Tin)
Sweet Corn	1.30	300(Tin)
Red Pepper	1.80	3
Flavours	1.30	Various
Sea or River Salt Flakes		
Total	11.75	

14 meals or soups	84 pence per meal	450 ml container per meal just add purified water & boil or liquidise into a soup

To make this meal with organic chicken, the cost is around £1.25 per 450ml container (2016)

Free video – go to www.utube.com search for Chemicalism

COOKING THE ORGANIC VEGEATBLES IMMEDIATLY IN A PRESSURE OR AIR SEALED COOKER AFTER PURCHASE PROVIDES THE HIGHEST NUTRITION

FREEZING THE ORGANIC MEALS LOCKS IN THE NUTRITION OF YOUR FAVOURITE TASTING READY MEALS

Enjoyable Flavouring is essential for a natural nutrition lifestyle

The flavourings can be made in different ways from natural products such as garlic, Thai lemon grass, herbs, spices, natural salt. With a busy work life, I have turned to a handful of organic stock cubes with these flavours.

Tomato and Herb
Mushroom
Garlic and Herb
Chicken
Vegetable
Beef
Vegetable
Curry Powders
Chili Powder

Making the meals look attractive with the colourful vegetables on the top adds to the appetite because we eat with our eyes first in many cases.

Chem

STEP 2

A leap of faith with courage to take action in a new direction

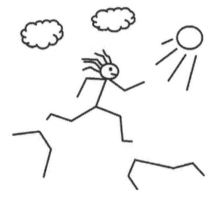

"Courage is what it takes to stand up and speak; courage is also what it takes to sit down and listen."

Winston Churchill

"Efforts and courage are not enough without purpose and direction."

John F. Kennedy

"The opposite for courage is not cowardice, it is conformity. Even a dead fish can go with the flow."

Jim Hightower

"Inaction breeds doubt and fear. Action breeds confidence and courage. If you want to conquer fear, do not sit home and think about it. Go out and get busy."

Dale Carnegie

Having accepted step one, you now need to take a big leap of faith and courage to believe a change in attitude will bring a good outcome for your healthy lifestyle.

Consider a thirty day fun boot camp approach. One organic meal and snack every day for thirty days. Step one was about preparation. Most people are able to succeed with a thirty day goal.

Just start the thirty habit today and let the rest of the days fall into place. If you have a gap in the thirty days it probably means you need more preparation time. Keep calm and carry on.

One organic meal and one natural snack along with the other foods you normally eat starts to build up a new lifestyle. It is unlikely anyone would change from a chemaholic to a natural nutrition lifestyle overnight. There is a lot to learn and experience to build up. These steps follow a logical path which is based on a proven method of recovery.

Taking a relaxed approach to your new lifestyle change deciding it will be easy and fun will help make it easy and fun! Even when with lots of un-wellness making a start is the only way to discover the benefits.

There is no need to explain to anyone about your change in attitude regarding swapping old values about nutrition for new better ones. This avoids the possibility of getting unhelpful comments. Avoid setting yourself up to be criticised heavily before getting started.

There is no need to people-please because your body and mind need looking after first.

People pleasing one or lots of people usually means putting yourself last in the queue, tired out and often not pleasing everyone. To be useful to others, you have to put yourself first at times.

The 12 steps will only make sense having experienced completing them during several weeks. Just like many subjects there is a logical building of knowledge. For example to write a sentence in a foreign language starts with learning the new alphabet. This book is more like a pocket size phase book to get you started without information overload!

To have an in depth knowledge of nature requires a lot of studying. There are one day courses to increase knowledge. To become qualified as a Naturopathic Therapist or Doctor it is possible through the professional organisations.

Many people have changed to proper natural foods before, so there is no need to argue or debate the subject of Chemicalism. All you want is your big share of a healthier lifestyle. Yes, it will take a few weeks to see results. The body is adjusting naturally, which is the best way for long term results.

Food gossip wastes time. Having a big open mind about consuming natural nutrition without artificial chemicals definitely means avoiding arguments. There is no need to argue with yourself about old unhelpful beliefs or other people about the truth of a food source. Just work with and seek out the facts as best available.

Nutrition value is the most important value

Having faith in natural food nutrition to provide good health is how the human race has been able to survive.

Many animal and fish species are becoming extinct due to modern day commercial influences or toxins entering their food chain. The world bee population is in decline.

Human beings experience premature deaths from increasing modern day ill health, especially obesity related.

People can avoid being influenced strongly by advertising messages by being aware of them and any kind of low price promotions.

Ask more questions

Ask yourself about the source of the food so you are responsible for the decision of what you decide to consume. Where does it come from?

Ask yourself about its growth and method of transportation from the source to your mouth.

Natural high nutrition foods are free of large amounts of artificial chemicals or contaminants, so the body is able to function better naturally because it does not need to struggle with processing unnatural chemicals.

Having a questioning approach from now on is essential! At the back of this book are some fun quick quiz question and answers.

These are examples of the questions you need answered as you evaluate what food nutrition you consume every day and then through new awareness choose the most natural options. Some of the answers are easy to see. For example if a vegetable or fruit does not state "Organic" then it is reasonable to believe it has artificial chemicals added.

A few moments of thought before you buy and eat makes a big difference.

Vegetables and fruit

- Genetically modified or organic?
- Sprayed with insecticide, pesticide? (Organic or non organic)
- Washed - boiled with tap water containing a range of weed killing chemicals?
- Altered by tap water added chemicals killing various bacteria – what is the list? (or purified) Check with your local water supplier.

- Tainted by pipes containing contaminates – lead – rust - other?

- Stored too long: how many hours, days, weeks, months how old is the source?

The word "cide" in Latin means "killer," "act of killing homicide " and is used in the formation of compounds pesticide, insecticide.

Vegetables

The base meal in step one is an easy start, low cost, high nutrition meal. Made in batches and frozen for convenience. There are many organic flavours you can add. This depends on your taste buds. Organic flavours are available as stock cubes.

Organic vegetables have an "organic" marked label in the supermarkets. This means the farmer is licensed to produce the organic product. The product will not be treated with chemicals to kill bacteria or insects.

Bacteria and insects cannot live on vegetables or fruits sprayed with chemical poison.

Two products that I usually pay almost double the price for are carrots and celery. However as both these organic products at full price cost under £1. They are already low cost. I enjoy them as snacks with organic houmous.

Fruit Bowl

One of my first new habits was simply having a working fruit bowl. This meant I had an easy way to grab snacks within seconds of feeling a strong craving to eat. The fruit is organic. Friends who grow their own apples have been happy to give me some of their surplus. Getting fruit from your own known natural sources is an example of when you will not packaging stating organic.

I used to believe organic fruit was too expensive with no health benefit. I did not know my friends had apple trees. I used to buy the fruit grown with pesticide; often wasting a percentage as it became out of date; hidden in the fridge.

Overall look at how to save money and reduce eating chemicals.

Fruit bowls can look like ornaments. The attractiveness helps create an enjoyable appetite for fast fruit food. Fruit contains natural sugar for energy. Enjoy having a fun fruit bowl and offer others a quick snack too.

Snacks and crisps

Fruit is a low cost snack; for example a bag of six organic apples may provide six snacks costing around the same price as two small bags of crisps.

Nuts are easy to nibble on. They can be organic.

Keeping them in a resealed container makes them easy to snack on when travelling.

Some crisp style snacks have less than 50% potato content. This means legally the manufactures do not have to charge VAT because the product is not legally a crisp. It can be called a snack and not be a crisp.

I enjoy crisps and snacks but prefer the brands with NO:

- MSG
- Preservatives
- Artificial colours

Baked products which may be classified as snacks usually have lower fat which sounds good to me.

These products are very tempting and often on sale in shops close to the checkout till for impulse purchasing.

Manufacturers have good websites showing all the ingredients and often have a free customer service helpline. Spending a few minutes to ask questions is another minor investment in personal health awareness.

The crisps I would most prefer are homemade. Sliced thin organic potatoes fried in coconut oil with sea salt. However, I am often too busy to make crisps. I enjoy buying them as one of my 20% low nutrition foods.

Appetite

To keep my chewing appetite satisfied I aim to keep listening for the signals. Chewing gum, crunching on raw fruit and vegetables plus spending more time chewing food helps satisfy my appetite. There are many factors that stimulate appetite including emotions and medications. When I get hungry the first thought is why?

Knowing how and when your appetite is triggered also means being able to prepare better snack and meal options.

Meat and Fish

Where did the fish grow up in natural water or a fish farm alternative?

Are the animals fed growth hormones?

What artificial chemicals have been introduced into the final product shown on the packaging?

The answer to some of these questions may not be on the packet. It may be answered by the super markets customer services helpline. This is step two and more answers will follow in other steps.

The price of organic meat and fish is often higher at first glance. This may be different if you are aware of the times in the day when supermarkets mark down prices due to sell by dates.

Save money when buying organic products by comparing the big differences on savings in the main supermarkets especially if you enjoy meat and fish. (see web links in appendix)

One lazy approach is to use a super market comparison website allowing you to upload your loyalty card details so it knows your food choices. Starting a new loyalty card for natural food and drink will increase the chances of supermarkets giving you discounts on those products. Supermarkets want to sell more. Bulk discount offers are worth having for the natural products you enjoy. Cook and freeze to lock in the nutrition.

Saving money is not important for everyone especially when a life threatening illness or health condition is the first priority.

There are many supermarkets and organic based meal companies that offer home delivery.

Fish is free to catch from the sea and we are on an island. The U.K. exports a lot of fish abroad. The U.K. imports a lot of fish from countries where it is cheaper to catch it.

I love to go to the seaside to eat fish and chips. I used to assume the fish came from the nearby coast but it is worth asking. The main thing is to enjoy the food and ask for any options. For example many fish and chip restaurants also offer grilled or poached fish.

Restaurant and fast food takeaway meals

These meals are unlikely to use non organic products so I treat these within my 20% allowance of low nutrition foods. I would rather not know what ingredients go into the meals in case it spoils my enjoyment.

Eating slowly helps me to listen to my body for any intolerant signs. However if I am drinking a glass of red wine my awareness of my body, gut reactions goes down.

The gut is so clever with informing the brain when it is not happy. It holds about 90% of the body's serotonin which influences our happiness levels. The brain holds less than 5% of serotonin. I think of the gut as an independent workforce. When the workforce is made unhappy it reacts by sabotaging the body systems it controls.

Water

Purified water is essential to the body; this must

be in place for good health to have a fighting chance as the number one priority.

There are different options to achieve 99 % + purified water. The easiest one is a hand held bottle available online or usually available from good camping shops. Ensure that it states the 99% purification of water as there are many cheap filters that only take out minor contaminates.

By producing your own purified water with better quality than unfiltered tap water it means saving money and time not having to buy bottled water.

Salt Butter Cooking Oil

The natural options are easy to find in the larger super stores. Salt is labelled as natural sea or rock salt. It tastes better so I use less.

Butter is marked as organic salted or unsalted. Using or spreading slightly less will probably make little difference to the money spent on butter. Using the natural butter assists weight loss if this is important. Margarine is not generally considered a natural product so check the ingredients to be sure of your choice.

Cooking Oil has many flavours. I enjoy coconut oil as I like the taste and the very high cooking temperature for a fast stir fry. This makes my washing up easy as well using only hot water.

There are many flavours of natural cooking oils to choose from. They do tend to be more expensive but by using slightly less it may not be a big difference in a monthly food budget.

These are small important changes to start ambushing your personal health improvements.

Thirty meals in thirty days

Thirty Organic meals in thirty days, one per day as the main meal: there are thousands to choose from. Importantly, eat foods other foods that you enjoy; they could be your new or old favourites. You may have three meals a day just have one of them as your organic meal so your lifestyle and body adjusts.

Chapter one has a simple low cost base meal to start. With a base meal you are able to add extra flavour, organic foods or change presentation when you are ready to eat.

Just start today working towards enjoying 70 – 80 % high natural nutrition with organic foods when possible. Make up the rest with some low nutrition products. Consider incorporating the many gluten free and wheat free options. This is not a cook book. A good book is listed at the back.

Low nutrition typically is:

- Food processed with artificial chemicals
- Fast food takeaway
- Mass produced low price ready meals
- Cheap white bread products
- Alcoholic drinks
- Non fresh – non organic fruit and vegetables
- Anything where there is very little trace of nature being the original source of its making

Enjoy it and smile, knowing you are looking after your general health with the 70 - 80 % high nutrition foods but without feeling deprived.

Being happy with a smile contributes to physical wellbeing.

Eating low nutrition foods slowly increases the nutrition value. Australian Koala's who are also mammals eat only very low nutrition food. They spend most of their non sleeping time chewing eucalyptus tree leaves.

There are many gluten free products which avoid containing a high cocktail of artificial chemicals and provide a good off the shelf (mail order) alternative initially for cakes, biscuits, cereals, chocolate. The main thing is to search for the products and ask questions about the source.

ısts

My approach has simply been to enjoy it, swapping to alternatives without artificial chemicals. I used to mix up every morning for over ten years a healthy labelled weight loss drink listing vitamins and minerals. However, I now understand this mix was packed full of artificial chemicals with sugar fuelling my obesity.

Today I enjoy gluten free cornflakes, chopped nuts, full fat organic milk, organic fruit, and usually warm water with fresh lemon. Sometimes I make up a liquidised drink with organic fruit and vegetables. My mum has enjoyed organic porridge then often later in the morning organic egg and bacon fried in coconut oil with gluten free toasted bread. There are many natural cooking oils to choose from and I look forward to tasting more.

Withdrawal

With the mental highs of a chemaholic, it is best to withdraw gradually, reducing physical and mental cravings. I changed from a 25 year habit of consuming artificial chemical sweeteners to Demerara brown sugar. This reduced my weight but my energy levels noticeably went down for two weeks.

Doing one major change at a time means it is

easier to monitor any withdrawal. My body needs convincing I have made the right change. Just the same as a sceptical, helpful, friend who needs to see the results before accepting the new truth.

In the first few weeks, my weight did increase slightly. This was scary. However, I felt confident high nutrition food was more important to focus on and not weight loss. Also, I had very sweaty armpits for about two weeks which I now understand was due to a new healthy level of detoxing.

Binge eating

Having long periods between snacks and meals increases the desire to binge, so having regular food breaks reduces strong cravings. Once the body is registering large reductions of something it has become used to. The mind starts wanting to return to what it had been taught was acceptable.

My experience of the "chemaholic high" after a long period without a "high" is very mentally rewarding, even though the body may complain physically afterwards. Much like an alcoholic binge drinking session, it could be considered worth it.

I have found the side effects from small binges are not very noticeable because the majority of my nutrition is high. Therefore my body usually quickly processes unwanted toxins. As there is no need to have announced the beginning of a new healthy lifestyle at this stage, there is no one to criticise your learning progress. This is covered in step twelve bounce back tests.

Exercise

This is secondary to the importance of consuming high nutrition food (unless a medical condition exists). The improved nutrition leads to more natural energy, stimulating an increased desire for exercise.

Phasing out Chemicalism is likely to coincide with a change in energy levels. Everyone is slightly different. Having some exercise everyday maintains good circulation, so it is good for everyone to enjoy some kind of exercise. It also stimulates chemicals in the brain to enhance mood, which is all good for coping with stress.

However it is possible; start today with some noticeable extra amount of exercise at this step. Here are some suggestions:

- Lifting your legs if you cannot walk
- Stretching your fingers if you arms cannot lift
- Parking your car further away to encourage extra walking

- If you are fortunate enough to have the ability to walk, swim, cycle, exercise for sport, use a leisure centre then give yourself a casual appointment to do so. Start with Ten minutes of new exercise.

The trick with getting started in any small way is just build an easy new habit into your new lifestyle. Then be happy with your new habit however small because it is the starting now that is most important.

Fake it to make it

I believe my mind often needs to see results before believing in them and has to be convinced visually. When I started to walk again after years of acute disabling back pain my exercise improvements were very slow. To be walking again pain free was amazing because orthopaedic consultants said this was not possible.

Whilst living mainly in a laid down position to reduce pain I visualised being young again driving a motorbike. Within a month of walking I saw the exact make and model of motorbike for sale that I used to drive. It was early days in my walking recovery so driving a motorbike seemed impossible. It was free to look! The owner offered me monthly payments. At first it seemed a crazy idea. Then I realised it was possible to drive this motorbike because it relied upon my balance not strength.

My mind found a way overnight to overcome my fears using the "fake it to make it" method. The bike's side stand allowed me to slowly tilt the bike into a start or park position. After I purchased the bike it was parked outside my front door just for motivation. It worked! Later I made many long journeys on that motorbike touring around The U.K. and France.

Taking one step in the right direction is how every marathon runner starts.

Medications

The modern day pill taking society offers a lot of choices. Many non natural options have side effects, including altering mood, weight, digestion, sleep pattern, energy during the day, liver function, and appetite. These side effects are mainly published by the drug manufacturer. Being sure of which side effects are resulting from the drugs is helpful to identify exactly what is making your body suffer.

Often natural alternatives are available by searching online, talking with knowledgeable staff in a health shop or a qualified naturopath. There are many physical side effects of Chemicalism which again are published. As more natural nutrition is absorbed into your body, it may become clear it is time to review medication.

In some cases, medications may require dosage adjustment, particularly if the original medical condition no longer exists, e.g. high cholesterol. It is good to review with a doctor or a medically trained person, and if possible to seek a second opinion from a naturopathic professional.

This is another area of potential money savings from:

- Purchasing the prescriptions
- Medicines to counteract side effects of prescriptions
- Time to attend and arrange medical appointments
- Cost of travel and time to obtain medications

This may also be a chaotic and stressful part of a lifestyle which may be reduced with improved health.

Take Action today to start the benefits

Getting started today with any extra improvements is more important than working on a perfect plan for tomorrow. Waiting for perfect conditions for starting is an easy disabling obstacle that is overcome with immediate action.

This book is deliberately short to increase the chances for an easy start.

Some people may decide they cannot start until they have finished reading the whole book. Often with self development it involves dabbling with new ideas before following a plan.

Please consider this book like a quick foreign language phase book:

- A logical method to pull together the steps
- Requires a big open mind to learn new values
- The basics need to be in place to get started on stage five
- Progress is better than perfection
- Only by using the steps may a long-term worthwhile meaning result

After completing the twelve steps, keep reviewing each step and enjoy a deeper understanding in a healthy lifestyle.

However, it may suit people to just start immediately, read a step, take action, complete the step then read the next step.

Motivation

I suggest to start believing and visualising an end goal to increase motivation if the goal is weight loss, then finding smaller size clothes to look forward to wearing and keeping them visible; these actions will help the mind focus.

Step two goals include motivation for better health to enjoy a favourite place with certain people, or to do a type of activity. Just start deciding what you are getting ready to enjoy with your improved health.

Consider regularly looking at pictures of what you are predicting. Perhaps put up a picture when you were many years younger, so the mind starts working on how the details can be worked out. I found a favourite picture of myself at twenty years old when I back packed around Europe for a month. This became framed and a reminder of my once good health.

Thinking takes time

It took me several weeks to find out how organic; natural food, drink and snack nutrition costs less than chemaholic options. This requires extra thought to discover new options using a new open minded approach.

It has not always been possible for me to find organic foods at a lower price or cost free because I like to travel. However, by aiming for high nutrition products when available my health has improved.

My investment with taking extra time to think through how it is possible to get hold of natural high nutrition foods has paid healthy dividends.

Take extra time to research the lower cost options for natural nutrition to improve both health and wealth.

Summary. Chemicalism Nutritional Quadrant

High Natural Nutrition No Chemicals (e.g. Organic Foods, Sunlight)	High Nutrition With Chemicals (e.g. vitamin, mineral supplements, filtered 99% drinking water)
Medium Nutrition With Chemicals (e.g. Gluten free, low level of chemicals, GM vegetables sprayed with pesticide)	Low Nutrition Chemaholic All or high Chemical content Highly processed, low or no natural content (e.g. potato snacks with less than 50% potato, non organic vegetables, unfiltered mains tap water)

In the above quadrant by Simon Kadwill-Kelly

*Chemical meaning manmade chemicals
*Chemaholic meaning low nutrition and high manmade chemical content

- Step two is a thirty day plan

- Eat one organic meal each day along with other meals

- Eat one natural food based snack each day along with other snacks

- Adopt this new value "Nutrition value is the most important value"

- Ask new questions about the natural origin of the food you eat

- List all your favourite foods and drinks on your personal menu

- Begin looking forward to an improved lifestyle with more options

- Listening better to appetite triggers

- Get a blood test after thirty days and discuss the results with a health professional

STEP 3
Trust In Nature
it really works

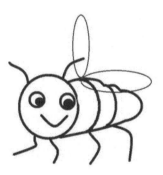

"Let food be thy medicine and medicine be thy food."

Hippocrates A Greek physician

Trust in anything or anyone new involves judging the benefits of the likely outcome.

"Natural" as a term used to sell products is unclear and has different legal meanings in different countries."Organic" is the most reliable term in the UK and does vary in other countries.

When I decided to trust in eating natural foods my friend Elsa gave me confidence. I was impressed that she had just passed a fitness test for a large chain of UK leisure centres as a personal fitness trainer.

I felt confident whatever the natural food lifestyle she followed was serving her well. I was also intrigued to find out how Elsa effortlessly kept slim with lots of energy to fearlessly enjoy sports, including roller blading around the streets of London.

Elsa's son, Adam, now 42, brought up since his birth on Nature Cure, is a very fit man. He continues with the lifestyle he is accustomed to. Adam never puts on weight and just like his mother. He hardly ever suffers illness except for minor colds that he shakes off within a couple of days. Adam travels the world using only high nutrition food for immunity and   medication.

Being open minded to change my attitude, change my beliefs about food to trust in nature like never before has been essential to my recovery from years of obesity.

Most of the advertising for food and drinks I was consuming before 2013 promoted healthy ingredients with likely outcomes of weight loss, more energy and generally better health. Trusting the advertising gave me very strong beliefs about nutrition that I was doing the best for my health. However, my lifestyle was suffering as I became more obese.

Elsa had followed a lifetime lifestyle based on Naturopathy, which is an over 200-year-old alternative medicine standing the test of time. Naturopathy is used to treat or prevent (through immunity) diseases without the use of drugs, by using diet, exercise, and massage techniques. I already believed in osteopathy and homeopathy for curing my back pains. These treatments come within the natural healing techniques of Naturopathy.

The food and drinks I was consuming contained a high level of unnatural (artificial) chemicals that confused my body as it attempted to process, store, and treat some of them as toxins. This low nutrition caused me to binge eat.

This triggered neurotransmitters in my brain to crave food to raise and settle my happiness levels. This addiction was very tiring because I felt afraid to eat in case I put on more weight. I was addicted to consume artificial chemicals in food to reduce stress. I started introducing more natural organic foods whilst reducing the artificial chemicals to a low level.

My solution of consuming about 80% natural high nutrition foods is working well because I am not feeling deprived of any food I want to eat.

There are many situations at work when the only food options are consuming low nutrition products. My body is better able to filter the artificial chemicals.

Three supplements that I believe support absorbing nutrition better and maximise natural energy are:

- Amino acids
- Q10 (Co-Q10 co-enzyme)
- Probiotics

My mum's immunity at 94 years increased through eating a high percentage of natural, organic food, a change which led to her recovery from gangrene and reduction in cholesterol to normal levels in 2014. This convinced me further that eating mainly natural food allows the body to work better with fighting dis–ease.

I no longer get weeks of cold and flu symptoms every year, automatically with a chest infection needing two courses of antibiotics to cure it. Nowadays I occasionally get a cold, it usually goes away quickly by using natural remedies which often cure it sometimes in less than a 24 hours. This all saves money on lots of medicines I used to buy but most of all I am not wasting my life away suffering from illness.

Mankind has been successful at surviving on this planet for thousands of years by consuming locally sourced, natural food products. Now we have developed:

- International transportation systems with freight containers to move food long distances

- Make food products low cost by using low cost labour and economic advantages around the world

- Mass food production manufacturing processes using artificial chemicals

- Large superstores encourage higher consumer purchasing volumes

- Brands are promoted through dynamic marketing techniques

The local supply of food has mainly been swapped for a much wider range of internationally distributed low cost foods. This has allowed more low nutrition foods to be consumed.

Oxygen

A natural oxygen supply gained through high nutrition foods is essential for wellbeing and healing. Oxygen travels around the body in the blood stream.

When the blood supply gets clogged up or slowed down too much, restricting the oxygen supply, all kinds of unhealthy conditions are given an opportunity to begin, for example, gangrene.

My mum (aged 93 yrs) first changed to a natural food lifestyle in 2013; I believe her oxygen supply increased through natural foods. This explains why my mum's terminal gangrene in both feet became naturally healed in 2014. The standard cure offered to my mum was amputation of the gangrene leg, but my mum said "No"!

When I was obese, a numb feeling of "pins & needles" at the ends of my fingers and toes had become normal after a night of sleep. This sensation I believed was due to a lack of exercise in my busy lifestyle. After a few weeks of my new lifestyle the pins and needles disappeared.

Mum's enthusiasm about her recovery increased with her revived belief in many natural herbs, such as ginger and garlic. She was taught about herbs as a child by her grandma. My mum developed a renewed love for tasty foods, including Manuka Honey in her porridge every morning. My mum said food had become much more tasty. I agree this is one of the rewarding benefits from eating lots of natural foods.

There were many natural cures through nutrition that my mum used, and to speed up recovery. Mum used a simple electric circulation booster gadget each day. The combined effects meant mum was able to get her fingers working again and enjoy chopping up vegetables. Mum created her own recipe of organic ready meals which we would make together in batches then freeze them to lock in the nutrition.

My mum's appetite was smaller compared with my own. This meant my homemade meals have been frozen in 450ml containers and mums in 200ml. This avoided wastage and halved the cost of my mum's meals to about 40p! However, nutrition is the most important value.

When mum had acupuncture for the first time in 2014, she really enjoyed it. At that stage of her path toward wellness, the gangrene had completely been cured by September 2014. Mum had gained a new sense of courage, extra mental agility, a more open mind, and greater interest in learning about natural healing. This is exactly what has happened to me and many people who are following this lifestyle change step by step.

Mum surprised nurses, doctors and consultants at how, aged 94yrs, she had recovered from so many illnesses within about six months of a new high nutrition lifestyle. My mum hoped to inspire other people to follow her recovery through her short book. She proudly overcame her terminal gangrene and said "No" to a leg amputation and also recovered from years of diabetes type II.

Being an essential part of nature, honey bees produce honey that can be used for so many remedies. With many healing properties, Manuka honey from New Zealand is considered one of the very best. Bees have been a puzzle to scientists for a long time. In theory, a creature should not be able to carry the same weight as its own body weight. Bees actually should be too heavy to fly, especially with their small wings.

Trusting in nature in this step simply means returning to what we human beings and animals were naturally designed for.

Most people believe they are eating food that is

close to nature as they trust in the packaging, the methods of promotion. People are puzzled why they are not enjoying a healthy lifestyle with an average weight. This is understandable because the media does an excellent job with promoting products to the most profitable mass market.

There is a growing number of people changing to trusting in natural products. This can be noticed with the large super markets offering more natural products, many having an organic, whole foods and a gluten free section.

Digesting Vegetables

I do not consider myself a vegetarian. However, after some short research it turns out human beings have similar physical characteristics to animals with plant based nutrition.

Human beings since thousands of years ago lived on plant based foods. Our close relatives in the animal world are gorillas and chimpanzees which are vegetarian with similar canine teeth.

Meat eaters generally have claws or fangs. They automatically salivate when seeing another living animal such as when a cat sees a mouse or raw meat.

To hide the taste of fresh blood and flesh it is cooked and flavours added.

Since thousands of years ago humans have become clever by making tools and technology. The use of these has widened our diets to include flesh and fish.

The stomach acid needed inside a natural meet eating animal is high enough to digest tough animal tissue, bones. Also handle the cholesterol in the meat.

Vegetarian creatures have long digestive intestines and if they eat meat it is important to have extra fibre to get rid of the flesh foods. Meat eating animals have short intestines to quickly digest flesh and blood.

Perspiration through the skin is normal for a vegetarian but meat eaters perspire through the tongue.

These facts maybe of more interest to anyone researching about their own digestion un-wellness.

One of Britain's fastest growing lifestyle trends 2016

News, 17 May, 2016

There are three and half times as many vegans as there were in 2006, making it the fastest growing lifestyle movement

There are over half a million vegans in Britain - at least 1.05% of the 15 and over population* - new research commissioned by The Vegan Society in partnership with Vegan Life magazine, has found.

At least 542,000 people in Britain are now following a vegan diet and never consume any animal products including meat, fish, milk, cheese, eggs and honey. This is a whopping increase since the last estimate of 150,000 ten years ago, making veganism one of Britain's fastest growing lifestyle movements.

The study, carried out by leading researchers Ipsos MORI, surveyed almost 10,000 people aged 15 or over across England, Scotland and Wales – the biggest ever poll quantifying the vegan community.

"To have over half a million vegans in Britain is fantastic.

More people than ever before are acting upon the health and environmental benefits of veganism, and finding out what really goes on in the meat and dairy industries and deciding they do not want to contribute to the pain and suffering of animals," said Jasmijn de Boo, CEO of The Vegan Society.

The results make encouraging reading for those who care about animals and the planet. Nearly half of vegetarians who are not vegan said they would like to reduce their consumption of dietary animal products. This equates to 521,000 people across Britain, meaning there could soon be in excess of one million vegans in total.

The movement is being driven by young people making more ethical and compassionate choices – close to half of all vegans are in the 15-34 age category (42%) compared to just 14% who are over 65 – evidence to support even greater growth in the future.

The study also found that 3.25% of the population, around 1.68 million people, are either vegetarian or vegan. More than 860,000 of all vegetarians and vegans also avoid all non-dietary animal products such as leather and wool.

The vast majority of vegans live in urban or suburban areas (88%) compared with rural areas (12%) and this is reflected in London, where 22% of all vegans in Britain live – more than any other region.

Vegan Life magazine publishing director Keith Coomber said: "The public perception of veganism is changing fast. It's no longer an extreme lifestyle, it's easy and accessible - you can walk into any supermarket and be greeted by a huge range of dairy-free milks and many more other vegan-friendly products.

"As consumers become more savvy about the reality of the farming industry, and the health implications of meat and dairy products, this boom will only continue."

De Boo added: "The reasons behind the rise of veganism are numerous: the positive portrayal in the media has contributed to its changing image; documentaries on the shocking realities and consequences of animal agriculture have gained prominence; delicious-looking vegan recipes have multiplied online and on social media as society becomes increasingly health-conscious; and top vegan athletes keep proving that you can be fit and healthy on a plant-based diet.

Thank you to The Vegan Society for permission to reproduce this content. More information can be found at www.vegansociety.com

I am not suggesting becoming a vegetarian only that it is good to be aware of the latest trends in eating lifestyles.

Summary

- Natural nutrition for immunity and healing
- Review supplements
- Discover local supplies of natural foods
- Oxygen in the body is important for best health
- Say "No" to ill health
- Be aware why people are eating more vegetables
- WONDEA

STEP 4

List and search for a nutritional SPRING CLEAN!

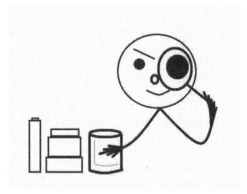

"The way to get started is to quit talking and begin doing."

Walt Disney

Making a deep, searching, thorough inventory of my food, drinks and chemicals I was consuming and then having a spring clean sounds simple. However, it took me several weeks to let go of old beliefs first whilst learning more about reducing low nutrition products.

Food is money

My belief had been so strong all my life that food is like money and should not to be wasted. In 2013, it was the first time in my life when I concluded that too much low nutrition foods with artificial chemicals were:

- Costing me more financially in poor health with having time off work

- Wasting excessive time visiting my doctor

- Using up time and money collecting prescriptions

- Having to buy supplements to top up my low nutrition

- Reducing my energy to enjoy leisure time

My old belief about not wasting foodslowed down my spring cleaning a lot.I found it difficult to give away or throw away foods that I had paid for, even though the artificial chemicals in them were not in agreement with my new healthy lifestyle.

People are starving

Wasting food or leaving part of a meal I associated with the strong belief that I had to eat it because there are starving people in the world. To overcome this guilt, I gave a lot of tinned foods each week to a homeless gentleman who sells the big issue close to my home. He was grateful, and I was thankful. I had stock piled a lot of tinned products. Throwing away the out of date ones was the easiest part.

There are many small local food distribution charities that are grateful for donations of food and will often collect.

Withdrawal

I slowly consumed the old lifestyle foods after I had introduced the new natural ones. It was a good plan to phase them out gradually. When I gave up artificial sweeteners overnight in exchange for brown sugar, I did experience an unexpected noticeable withdrawal. Most addiction recovery programmes encourage reduction first as a new lifestyle is put in place. This includes a new attitude to an addiction for a long term recovery.

List & advice

It took me about a month to review the many food products in my life, seeking advice along the way about the artificial chemicals. The more I threw away, the more I found to review, which turned into a valuable learning process. This encouraged me to make a list of the foods and chemicals in them to get advice about so I could keep checking what the natural alternatives would are.

Family – partner – sharing kitchen considerations

My friend who had been diagnosed with cancer was following a similar lifestyle change to save his life. He had decided to become cured by eating only natural ingredients without added sugar. His family did not fully understand his eating plan. He made the bold decision to have his own kitchen cupboard and eat separately to become cured with natural foods he enjoyed. Each time I look in the food cupboards, my eyes choose the menu options. I had to be sure the right products were in place.

Substitutes – Long term food storage

The home long term food store cupboard still has tinned foods which include:

- Organic soups
- Organic sweet corn
- Organic baked beans
- Organic lentils
- Organic tomatoes
- Fish in different flavours

There are many convenient organic options I keep stocked. These are for occasional use when I run out of fresh natural foods or need to grab something easy to heat up at work. These are usually more expensive. However I only use a very small amount compared with when I was a suffering chemaholic.

The many flavouring additives in the cupboard at the moment include:

- Organic flavouring cubes chicken - beef - vegetable
- Real lemon grass - garlic - chillies for stir frying
- Spices and herbs in powders - curries - tandoori - tikka-masala

- Organic tomato sauce to go with organic fried eggs

The amount of opened bottles of chemaholic sauces that used to be hidden at the back of the cupboards was embarrassing.

When I do choose a low nutrition meal or tinned option I usually top it up with something natural like chopped up organic celery.

Looking in my long term storage cupboard today it also includes:

- Porridge
- Gluten free cornflakes
- Organic soya milk – nut drinks - unopened cartoons
- Quinoa
- Brown rice
- Bottled beetroot
- Whole grain organic bread unopened airtight sealed
- Eggs
- Gluten free biscuits
- Manuka honey
- Organic Pasta

In the freezer it mainly stores frozen organic meals and also:

- Prawns
- Sausages
- Fish – different types
- Chicken
- Brussels Sprout
- Dark chocolate
- Ice cream

Having a healthier high nutrition lifestyle takes time to adjust to with finding the new options.

Store vouchers and points

Collecting shopping points at the main stores generated many special offer vouchers through the mail for products I no longer purchased. These vouchers are given based on regular purchases to encourage repeat or increased buying of the same. I started a new set of points cards with no history, and this has generated me many savings on the new natural foods. Also, I have points cards for health stores which have given me many savings. Eating before shopping encourages better judgement as it takes away the need for a fast food fix when the main priority is to purchase the products of high nutrition and best value.

Car – work – travel Bags

Snacks have always been on my list to keep stocked in different places. Knowing when and where snack cravings are likely to happen means that, with a small amount of preparation, natural food options can be in place. Places to include good snack options such as nuts and fruit include the car, draws at work, and travel bags. Anticipate your cravings. This should save money because snack purchases can be expensive. Especially where there are limited options such as at a motorway service station.

Cleaning chemicals

Chemicals enter the body from the outside of the skin in many ways. This is a good time to review the chemicals used in your washing up liquid that get mildly consumed into food and drink. The dishes, cups, pans, crockery, and cutlery may be washed with just hot water. Be mindful of the trace artificial chemicals from washing up liquid, which is then processed through your liver.

Some people use excessive washing up liquid. Once your taste buds become highly attuned again with natural foods, you may be surprised to start tasting the sour taste of washing up liquid.

There are natural alternatives for washing up liquid. Large super markets, often stock them next to brand name products. Research health shops and online stores with the many other natural household cleaning products. Checking prices and sizes makes it definitely possible to save money by buying washing up liquid based on natural ingredients.

The good news is that the skin reacts better to natural products. Over time you could save money on skin care products by using natural cleaning products. Skin is an organ, absorbing and reacting to whatever it is exposed to.

Some people already experience unwanted skin reactions from cleaning chemicals and need to buy rubber gloves just to do the washing up. Be aware of the chemicals absorbed into the skin. The liver has to filter a lot of modern day chemicals.

Consider treating your body to natural options with nutrition for hand soap, soap powder, and washing up liquid. Legislation for The EU has a newly created EU Chemicals Agency. "REACH," which stands for Registration, Evaluation and Authorisation of Chemicals. Registration will require companies to register information on chemicals by 2018. Washing up liquid will then start to become regulated.

The EU introduced "E" numbers in 1962 to define and regulate artificial chemical additives in food and drinks.

Cosmetics and skincare

Skincare, teeth, gum, shaving, hair products, skin washing products contain chemicals that get absorbed into the body. Be aware of what chemicals you are absorbing and consider natural alternatives. Smelling the natural ingredients you enjoy usually brings about an uplifting or relaxing mood change.

Being happy with different lifestyle improvements includes the smells we choose to use in products. Some natural cosmetics also have a healing ability. If you have skin conditions being treated with medication also consider natural alternative options. With any new healing product for skin you choose just try it on a small area for a few weeks to be sure it is the right choice.

There are thousands of natural options. Also be aware of any skin addiction withdrawal to medications especially hormone based ones.

My feet used to suffer regularly with a fungal infection called Athletes foot. (Inflammation between the toes.) I used a prescription cream for many years to keep killing the infection. This went away after I had lost 22 kilos by changing to more natural nutrition. I was surprised and wonder if the tea tree soap and manuka honey shampoo helped the healing. When my mum was treating a similar condition on her feet she used colloidal silver in a spray.

Medicines and supplements

It is a good idea to review medicines every few weeks with a doctor and or pharmacist in case they may require adjusting in the light of improved health and blood test results. Be aware of side effects from drugs from the manufacturers published information. Also there may be self help groups locally that offer support with giving up some types of drugs.

Chemical vitamins and minerals in tablet and powders may contain other chemicals or additives. These may not be required once swapped for natural, highly nutritious food.

First Aid Kits

When tidying up the bathroom make sure there is a ready to go first aid kit for emergency large skin wounds. If you drive a vehicle make sure there is a good first aid kit easy to grab in an accident. Ensure holiday travel items include large bandages. To have several large long bandages is essential for stopping artery wounds pumping out blood.

There is no cost consideration when it comes to saving a life from a big wound. Hospital and ambulances cannot be expected to respond quickly especially in bad weather or busy times.

The skin is our biggest organ to look after. When blood is pumped out from a severed artery or wrist a bandage is required within several minutes to avoid death. To have a good first aid kit may save an emergency hospital visit.

Rewarding

Keep spoiling yourself with new and more tasty meals and snacks to reinforce your new lifestyle. Taste buds work better after a few weeks of returning to a natural food lifestyle. Enjoy the foods you like and discover the natural alternatives. There are shows and fairs every year promoting an ever increasing amount of natural food options.

Decluttering helps make true the new "normal"

Before you announce your life style changes to yourself and others, "prove it by doing it." When people notice your change before you announce it, the chances of negative criticism from other people could be reduced because they cannot argue with what is now fact and history.

In spring cleaning the kitchen cupboards and starting to feel more mental energy from natural nutrition, this tidying up and reviewing life style may positively affect other areas of your life.

Reviewing my food cupboards, throwing many items away, or if I could not bear the thought of having thrown away something I paid for, using it up made space to see the good stuff left as well as the new good things.

A lifestyle change from an addiction recovery reveals more improvements with a feeling of revitalised energy. I started to de clutter with enthusiasm.

The perfectionist element can be disabling. There is no need to commit to the perfect moment to make a change, just make a small change that takes a few minutes. For example there was one draw in need of sorting out which I use first thing every morning. It took me 15 minutes. This small change saves me searching an extra 30 seconds to grab things each day. My morning feelings start with better clarity. This small improvement helps start my days with a feeling of happy organisation. Also I am getting an extra two hours of my life back per year!

Feeling good from high nutrition makes the brain work better, and eventually people will notice in different ways. Weight loss was the biggest one for me. I painted the walls fresh colours, got different clothes, threw away, or gave away clothes to charity. I got a new duvet cover with a happy pattern.

All of these actions gave me a new energy in my new lifestyle. Reviewing and clearing the bathroom of the various medicines was much like the reviewing the kitchen cupboards. There were many things that were no longer needed, some out of date. Being more minimal improved my health by not seeing reminders of my past unwell lifestyle.

Reviewing each product, the cupboards and other places have been cleared out. My eyes confirm to the brain this is the new undisputed truth, reinforced every day. All the new knowledge about ingredients in the food cupboards made me understand better why I had been obese for so long. Replacing the chemaholic foods gradually with new natural high nutrition options has been an education.

The transition to eating tasty, chemical-free food created my new "normal". This new truth leads into step five with confidence.

Summary

- High nutrition overall saves money and time
- Foods for charity
- Withdrawal can be phased in
- Learn more about the artificial chemicals no longer required
- The skin is our biggest organ to look after
- Review medicines
- Long term food storage reorganise
- Declutter
- Blood test results ready for step five

STEP 5

Announce to yourself and others your new plan IS underway

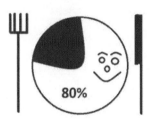

"Give me six hours to chop down a tree and I will spend the first four sharpening the axe."

Abraham Lincoln

Be proud to have changed many small parts of your life to enjoy the benefits today.

Up to this point, there has been no need to mention the choice to start a healthier lifestyle to anybody. The reason for this decision is to avoid unhelpful criticism that could stop progress on a new, life changing path without having given that lifestyle a chance to develop.

With step four completed, you will see the proof of your plan having been started with completed action. This is the new personal truth.

My own revelation, admission, and acceptance of overeating artificial chemical foods had been the big first step.

At this stage, you should have another blood test plus have a doctor or health professional check the many small adjustments in lifestyle habits that is your new "normal" to see if these changes have resulted in healthier medical records.

Confirmation of an improvement in health by a doctor qualified professional will be a big boost confidence. When you now encounter criticism, you will have a stronger, more relaxed response, knowing the facts in the improved health tests.

By step 12, it is possible you will have linked up with many new people who are living or working on healthier lifestyles. You may also find that some people who choose to lead an unhealthy lifestyle have become slightly more distant. The same unhealthy people may later value your inspiration. It is so important to keep aware of your journey and be thankful for the improvement.

People may have noticed a change in your appearance after several weeks. Steps one to four are about preparation. When people asked me what I was doing to look healthier, the easiest answer was to just say "eating more natural food." Most people did not really want a detailed answer unless they were so unwell and desperately ready for a change.

However, as I knew there was a lot more to learn, as there always is. My first suggestion to anyone wanting a change has usually been to have a go at making a batch of homemade, frozen, tasty, ready meals with organic ingredients.

Sometimes, I give away an easy recipe with the cost per meal worked out to show the money saved then see if the person is serious. This strategy has made me a few new friends. Importantly, it has kept me from chattering away about my new more enjoyable healthier life to people who are not prepared to take any kind of action towards theirs.

Some people hold on to their unhelpful nutrition values with a big grip, preferring to complain about their suffering. The big soul-searching question I asked myself at the beginning was "am I sick and tired enough of being sick and tired to change my lifestyle by trusting in nature?"

Looking and acting healthier often invites comments from suffering chemaholics. Beware they may just want someone to listen to their merry go round stories of chemaholic suffering. They may be interested to discuss how they were intending to start their changes towards enjoying a healthier lifestyle. Ill heath can be very confusing and a health diary is one way of starting to understand what is happening.

I understand it can be comforting to talk with fellow sufferers with empathy rather than sympathy. The important thing for me has been moving out of my comfort zone with an open mind to take action. It took me about six to eight weeks to prove the first results. The blood tests were facts which made me and others believe in natural nutrition with more confidence.

When I discovered eating full fat butter was

healthier than artificial chemical alternatives, I wanted to share this exciting knowledge with a friend. Unfortunately, she is a suffering chemaholic with diabetes type II. She responded with a strong argument about her chemaholic beliefs. This was based mainly on the packaging and advertising that claimed to promote a reduction in her cholesterol. The trust in her doctor had convinced her that her un-wellness was not reversible. She still believes the only solution to cope with her health conditions are to manage them with a cocktail of tablets three times a day. This belief was too strong to be challenged.

I used to cling to a lot of unhelpful beliefs when suffering with obesity and would argue my corner. Yet remain puzzled why my cholesterol continued to increase over years of being a suffering chemaholic? This is covered more in step 12.

Understanding the past better brings more freedom

Having a go at making a list about my old eating habits from memory as far back as could recall was a real help when admitting my old habits about Chemicalism to three trusted people individually.

Sharing many beliefs with three other healthy people was important to successfully make my new beliefs solid ones. Fortunately, I admitted all about my previous poor health to people with a proven healthy lifestyle.

They questioned me a bit which helped uncover a better understanding about some of my repetitive patterns. For example I used to go food shopping in the evening before having dinner this encouraged me to purchase more deserts and sweets to eat later. Now I still buy sweets and deserts for immediate consumption but after I have eaten dinner. This usually involves visiting a local shop which gives me a few paces of exercise.

Having reflected on what nature's high nutrition has on offer. I understood how I had become so unwell and obese. My new attitude towards nutrition helped me to identify many of my old habits which could be adapted to new, better habits. For example, I liked fast food meals, using a microwave at work and home. By making them myself with organic foods meant I had found a reliable way to work with one of my daily habits. Surrounding myself with natural food snacks and meals for convenience at work or away from home reduced my chemicalism.

This process felt very freeing with and all three people saying they enjoyed being trusted with my confidence in them. This is a humbling experience and takes a bit of effort to admit the details of past unhelpful habits.

One of the three people I had only ever known as being very slim and healthy. I was so surprised when she explained how she used to be very over weight and had to overcome many emotional eating disorder barriers which she was still working on. By me sharing my honest admissions it has given some people permission to allow them to share their experiences without fear of judgement.

I asked each one of these people who knew my story if they would guide me better on my journey and how they would do it. This open ended question proved very valuable, and I continue to learn with them.

Support from other healthy people

There are plenty of people who give me good advice at places where people are doing health-orientated activity, weight loss classes, swimming pools, and free health exhibitions.

Some people are just very good listeners, which is helpful when off loading thoughts, but I recommend seeking out knowledgeable, trustworthy people to inspire you onto the next step of better health.

A fewer number of people were happy to support

me a bit better with email/phone contact, which often has been a helpful two way exchange of ideas.

The best advice has come from a handful of people involved with personal coaching/health instructing in some way as a job (with a belief that natural foods are best.) They understand goals with clear stages are important when achieving a worthwhile plan.

This does not mean hiring an expensive personal trainer is essential. Often, short casual conversations with people living healthy lifestyles have been a very helpful ways to gain and swap valuable tips. I just encourage anyone to be open to having conversations with like-minded, health-orientated people to gain support and possibly make new friends.

Fortunately, I had found a new handful of fit people passionate about healthy eating who recognised I was open minded, receptive to acting on their good advice, and prepared to come out of my old comfort zone.

Health diary

If you have been hesitating to buy a separate health diary perhaps for fear someone may take fun then now is the time to get one as it is a good investment to see clear progress has happened with a plan in place.

Keeping a separate health diary to track progress is a valuable tool. I suggest getting one with a cover which brings a smile. Mine has a photo of me at 20 years old on it, looking fit and happy just before travelling around Europe for one month by trains.

Digital records are usually reliable but having a hard copy diary may be easier for some people like me. Having a paper based diary means you are able to doodle in it with a fun creative style. Immediately, I wrote in the first and second blood test results and once weekly weight recordings. This all helped raise my confidence should anyone criticise the facts.

Rewards are important especially using natural options

Natural pink Himalayan bath salts are a good way to relax, detox and absorb natural minerals through the skin. The skin is the largest organ. With announcing your plan this maybe a good time to start enjoying a new rewarding habit to increase your confidence of wellbeing.

Summary

- Feel confident with an improved health proven with facts

- Share the new knowledge with other people selectively

- Keep moving out of a comfort zone

- Understand better why old habits caused un-wellness

- Discover healthy people that support an improved wellbeing

- Enjoy talking and learning about a healthy lifestyle

- Have special natural rewards to strengthen the healing

STEP 6

Exchanging deprivation for ABUNDANCE

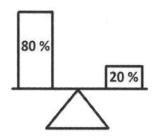

"Abundance grows with a bigger attitude of gratitude"

Swapping from low nutrition to high nutrition foods is a massive change in lifestyle and doing it gradually over several weeks makes it possible.

Celebrate! Consider having an organic food party or providing someone with an organic meal who is unwell. People on low nutrition lifestyles are often very surprised how good high nutrition foods taste.

Many people attempt a healthy lifestyle change with no preparation or long-term plan, making only small insignificant actions. I used to make regular attempts by eating a few more genetically modified vegetables. I now believe the insecticides and tap water chemicals had kept me unwell.

It is time to enjoy your new health, find new recipes, and experiment with new, natural ingredients.

Calorie burning

Low nutrition foods tend to burn off energy at a very slow rate compared with high nutrition foods that provide higher energy and burn off at a higher rate. Calorie counting does not incorporate the rate of how fast artificial chemicals take to burn off in my opinion.

After the first few weeks of switching to natural foods, I started to eat much more and continued losing weight. This was confusing at first because I used to believe in calorie counting. I was no longer afraid to eat lots of organic foods and this attitude has remained the same.

The foods I eat are more simple. I am grateful to have much better health with a higher amount of physical energy.

Calorie counting

This new way of lifestyle of being able to eat more quantity and quality of food was completely against all my previous beliefs. Counting calories is usually an inaccurate mental exercise, studies show most people underestimate.

The standard calorie consumption and burning off rates for an average person may vary a lot due to a person being:

• Shorter - taller

• More or less muscular

• Older – younger Suffers from a medical condition

• Uses weight altering medications

• Many other factors

The mass marketing of food products normally advertises counting calories rather than nutritional content.

I no longer count calories and have swapped that belief for aiming to enjoy tasty high nutrition foods. It is a lot easier to focus on nutrition content rather than calories.

Restock the kitchen cupboards, fridge, freezer

Having tasty natural foods in stock as options for my eyes to consider reduces my need to go elsewhere. This also saves money and time. What I enjoy best are many choices of foods with lots of flavours that are available within minutes, either hot or cold.

Takeaways, restaurant meals, fast food

My old fears about not eating foods which most conventional diets considered bad or naughty has now completely changed. I used to try to avoid these tasty foods considered too full of many ingredients that contribute towards obesity. (See bounce back tests.)

These type of meals I would regularly gulp down every week and almost happy to suffer the side effects of:

- Physically feeling bloated within half an hour
- Feeling guilty that I had over eaten something not good
- Indigestion
- Wind flatulence
- Bad breath
- Small amount of reflux repeating
- Loose bowels or constipation

It used to be my regular choice of nutrition, along with a few tablets to reduce the side effects.

Fast Food: bring it on!

Nowadays, I usually have one or two fast food, chemaholic-style, low nutrition meals each week and enjoy them with no noticeable side effects. However, as the taste of them has now become inferior to my natural options, the attraction towards them is very low.

By eating any food that takes my fancy, I avoid feeling deprived. Knowing I have given myself permission to consume low nutrition fast food has reduced my cravings for it.

I enjoy many brand name fast foods, but with a lot of extra chewing in the initial mouthfuls. This extra chewing time helps me be more mindful about the environment and listening to any strong body signals.

I used to believe that all the food that had been paid for needed to be eaten. That approach led to gulping down a meal after I was full. Nowadays I may buy a tasty pasty and happily enjoy consuming half. This strategy avoids or reduces bloating.

Chewing the initial mouthfuls into a pulp over a few minutes extracts as much flavour as possible and provides a period during which I can think consciously about how different nutrition can be enjoyed.

This extra chewing helps the food get digested better because the natural chemicals (enzymes) in the mouth enable better digestion.

The best fast foods are the natural ones

There are many snacks that are made with natural ingredients, and discovering them has encouraged me to enjoy cooking for fun; even after a hard day's work, I now find it relaxing to cook for 30 minutes. Usually cooking either significantly reduces or increases my appetite; either one is OK.

Snacks everywhere

I tend to plan for impulse snacking at work, in the car, on holidays and late night by making sure there is a healthy snack ready. Good options for travel include organic nuts and fruit.

Have a go at growing or keeping alive a plant

Organic vegetables are can be grown. Seeds are cheap, earth is free, rain water and sun makes your food. There are lots of additives to grow plants faster but they are not essential. This is ideal for someone with a garden. I have met many people who say organic vegetables are too expensive but they have a big garden, laid to grass with no plants. Super markets and garden centres sell both seeds and part grown plants. I feel growing a few herbs; plants and vegetables make their existence valuable. When I lived in a flat with no garden I just bought herbs in pots from the local supermarket. If the plant dies or the seeds do not grow it is a good time to learn how to do it better next time.

Needs must

Sometimes, for whatever reason, it is not possible to eat in a healthy way. Aim to keep high nutrition consumption to about 70 - 80% of the time.

Most people cope with the other times much better without any big side effects from artificial chemicals. I believe to help my body cope with some of the everyday toxins in food and drinks.

I feel it is good to consume a small amount of everyday toxins to maintain a strong immunity to their side effects.

Summary

- Calorie burning is different with natural foods Restock with higher nutrition foods

- Enjoy some chemaholic meals without big side effects

- Increase enjoyment of natural foods with better taste buds

STEP 7
Pleasure and Stress Triggers Balanced with Humility

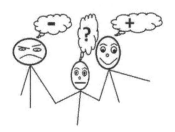

"Pride and vanity, the opposites of humility, can destroy our spiritual health as surely as a debilitating disease can destroy our physical health."
Joseph B. Wirthlin

"When someone saves your life and gives you life, there's gratitude, humility; there's a time you've been so blessed you realize you've been given another chance at life that maybe you did or didn't deserve."
Pat Summerall

"No one is immune from addiction, it afflicts people of all ages, races, classes, and professions."
Patrick J. Kennedy

"Our best thoughts come from others."
Ralph Waldo Emerson

I have sought many new ways to remove my controlling chemaholic lifestyle by altering my long term attitude and habits to gain extra humility.

Humbly admitting with true conviction I am a chemaholic. This meant leaving behind a familiar socially acceptable lifestyle of unhelpful beliefs about nutrition. To learn and practice a new lifestyle with an open mind took a big leap of faith.

Having lost excessive weight in six months, I over came many health conditions. Many people around me have died from unhealthy lifestyles or continue to suffer. I feel humbled, grateful to have been spared from a slow, suffering, premature death.

On 19th May 2008, my doctor broke the news I was diagnosed with cancer. My perspective of time changed overnight from believing I was going to die prematurely. Quickly prioritising a long to do list.

Then by deciding to give only real problems the expensive indulgence of attracting stress left only a small handful of tasks. Suddenly, most of my perceived high class problems that had previously been triggers to comfort eating chemaholic fast food were not stress-worthy.

The day after I was diagnosed with cancer, I got a parking ticket fine but decided it was no longer worth getting stressed about. Instead I wrote to the council for fun. Thanking them politely and asking them to kindly cancel it as I had not parked there before. The fun in finding the gratitude from previously stressful situations gave me more pleasure than the stress previously experienced.

I lost weight each week whilst believing I was going to die from cancer.

This shock made no difference to the types of food in my diet because I had no real understanding that I was a suffering chemaholic. Nobody mentioned that through diet, many people, including some published authors, have recovered from cancer. I did get better at handling stress by prioritising real problems which probably accounted for the reduced quantity of food I ate.

Previously, excessive stress was one of my triggers driving me to over eat as I believed such eating gave me a sense of short term stress release.

Several weeks after the initial diagnosis for cancer I had a second independent private hospital cancer test. This showed I did not have cancer. There had been a clerical typing error with the laboratory report which had been sent to my good doctor.

I started putting on weight afterwards, weight which increased every year until I introduced homemade organic meals in 2013.

Some high stress is healthy from time to time as we are designed to handle real, physiological, life-threatening problems. It is our natural basic instincts to get food and keep safe in a dry, warm shelter each day.

The majority of my life's previous problems were often not real life-threatening problems. These could have been reduced with a few, quick thoughts of gratitude and humility. This is what I have been taught and has served me well. I try not to get upset with small problems for example:

- A parcel or letter not turning up on time

- Software updates going wrong on my phone and computer

- Electrical products going wrong

- Waiting longer in an unexpected in a shop, on the phone or traffic jam

High stress reduced my immunity, so regularly getting colds or flu with a chest infection was normal. Instead of changing to natural food as a form of medicine. I would take lots of pills to keep on working on through being unwell, pills that would have put my body under extra strain.

The strain of working while being unwell fuelled my eating because I was desperate for extra energy. There were times when only an acute spinal pain due to all the inflammation stopped me from walking.

My body was telling me to rest but I did not pay attention. I was more convinced it was better to fight off the warning signals with medicines.

Both my feet had become extremely painful when walking due to the inflammation through obesity. I had wide fitting shoes with supports and spacers, but the toe bones were rubbing every day. This put me off walking; take more pain killers which fuelled my weight gain.

I was sick and tired of being sick and tired, suffering with aches and pains. However, I fortunately have had operations on both feet to get my bones back to their normal shape. Plus an operation on each shoulder. Now I enjoy walking, running, dancing, swimming and, most of all, cycling.

Most people know their own physical signs when they experience too much stress:

- Headache
- Neck ache
- Back ache
- Rashes
- Colds
- Tiredness
- Tremoring

There are so many over the counter medicines available to turn off or dull down our physical, natural, uncomfortable warning signs.

Naturopathy is about understanding the root cause of being unwell by taking account of the whole body to find a natural remedy.

I believe that if the brain has enough high nutrition, it is much better able to handle higher stress levels. Vitamin B is associated with improving the ability to cope with stress.

Everybody has their own stress boundaries, so it is good to keep testing out where these changing boundaries are. There needs to be some stress in life; otherwise, the boredom can be equally stressful such as part of the punishment of being locked up in prison.

Nowadays when faced with a choice between natural food options and a chemaholic ones. I quickly remember the physical suffering gone by; have thoughts of gratitude and choose to enjoy natural options.

Previously, my pride had kept me glued to a set of strong but incorrect nutrition beliefs. I was for over 30 years a suffering chemaholic on a tiring merry go round of expensive weight loss diets. Being proud of my incorrect knowledge about nutrition had stopped me from receiving advise.

My pride made my opinions about food rather defensive. These unhelpful opinions kept me obese and dictated my lifestyle with sources of unhealthy temptation. The sources of low nutrition food needed to change, and so did my pride. This change has often meant eating the most natural options alone avoiding trying to please people in social situations.

One of the reasons people tell me they cannot switch from a chemaholic lifestyle is by blaming their chemaholic family who would not tolerate a change. My married friend with three children handled this by gradually, secretly introducing natural nutrition each week. He told them two months later by explaining a camping holiday was the result of saving money on foods.

As a carer, I feel strongly that disabled, vulnerable and sick people deserve from their carer/s the best available natural foods to choose from. Create a quality lifestyle with maximum best health. Make people in your life the reason to enjoy natural, better health, not the excuse!

The less chemaholic food I ate and the more I digested my food better, the fewer the cravings and the happier my outlook has become.

Updating a separate food diary each day to understand the patterns can make the psychological triggers that cause a person to eat a lot from stress and pleasure usually become clear. There are so many personal triggers of stress: from seeing the mail unopened for fear of bad news, or perhaps feeling a lack of love in some way. Being addicted to anything that temporarily uplifts your feeling of happiness can be overcome by thinking of different ways to react.

Physical triggers of withdrawal maybe very strong, so by gradually changing to, enjoying more, and being surrounded by more natural high nutrition foods is the best long term approach. The mind has to fool the body.

My two very socially acceptable core addictions originated from being a workaholic and perfectionist, which I am aware of every day. Identifying the trigger to addictions, then working to erase or minimise those unsettled emotions is important to stop the many outward addictive behaviours, alcohol intoxication, smoking, gambling, taking drugs, eating badly.

One of the big times that people seek a "fix" from food is when they have a stressful day. It is one way of coping with stress. The stress happens anyway, so it is how we handle it that counts. At the end of a busy day, I love to take a bath with Himalayan bath salts, nourishing the skin, detoxing. Having a swim and sauna are other options to help with relaxing plus enhance sleep.

Some people get stressed with trying to control other people, places and things. This is mainly an impossible task. The only thing that is certain is everything changes.

Pleasure stimulation for all kinds of addictions, including sex, food, and alcohol, are triggered by the brain producing a rewarding chemical called "dopamine" which makes us feel happy. The dopamine released in the brain can be triggered by looking at pictures, smelling, and hearing, which all happen before consuming or experiencing the actual pleasure.

Some places, such as expensive hotels and restaurants, may make the experience exciting. The atmosphere also makes it easy to reduce awareness of the nutritional value of food you are eating. It is more difficult to judge the nutrition when there are no labels to read, so listening to your body's reaction is probably the best judge.

I like to enjoy the false, pleasurable glamour of the expected quality of food in a nice looking restaurant, knowing there is a fair chance of being served food with low nutritional value. Not feeling deprived is important. Nowadays when in a restaurant, I am able to stop eating low quality food half way through the meal. Eating slower is one way to better judge non labelled foods. It took several weeks before I truly valued nutrition more than consuming all the food for which I paid.

Getting pleasure from the smell of food cooking

can possibly give more pleasure than the actual consumption. Learning to like the smell of high nutrition foods has made it easy for me to switch mainly to them.

Being aware of this "dopamine fix" is helpful because as one lifestyle change is made to reduce an addictive "dopamine fix," another type of addictive behaviour is highly likely to become the next trigger.

When I gave up alcohol, my smoking increased. When I gave up smoking, my alcohol consumption increased. Finally, I gave up both on the same day. Then, I was overeating for a fix. For a while, this led to my over-exercising, being addicted to swimming and became a lifeguard. When realising what had happened, I decided to relax and study. The studying then took over whilst I was passing one or two I.T. exams per week and became qualified as an I.T. teacher in 2003.

It is very normal when someone overcomes their first major addiction that soon after, another addiction will take off. Therefore, getting to the root cause of the thoughts triggering the addiction is essential to handle the desire for a temporary, and false, uplift in mood.

When the pleasure chemicals (designed for essential survival instincts of sex and food) are artificially over-stimulated, the brain cleverly reduces the pleasure reward received, which means it takes a lot more stimulation to get the same natural "dopamine fix." It is understandable why eating low nutrition; tasty food may lead to requiring larger portions for the same pleasure to feel normal.

Heroin addicts always remember their first fixes as being the best highs. Once they are heavily addicted, the long term ongoing fixes are about just trying to feel normal to function. This is the usual way physical and behavioural addictions take over a person's life. Up to the mid 1950's, heroin in the U.K. was prescribed everyday to anyone for coughs, colds, diarrhoea, pain killing, and migraine headaches. It is a good example of how something that was considered good for many years has proven to not be thanks to reliable research.

There are many prescribed medicines designed to give patients an artificial way of generating more dopamine.

Rewarding myself with a holiday or a few hours without worrying about problems is very calming. Many problems are not real, genuine, life-threatening ones should be possible to dispel with humbling thoughts of gratitude.

Being given the news of suffering from a life-threatening health condition can be a brilliant starting point, for a change in attitude towards food being a medicine. This is especially true when other people have been cured from the same un wellness through natural medicine and high nutrition foods. (See recommended books.)

Keeping a health diary is a great tool for tracking habits and learning more about uncovering personal triggers. Once you feel you have overcome the chemaholic behaviour pattern that had a strong hold over your life, there may be another addiction that takes over—for example, over exercising to replace the desire for a mood change as a " fix", "high", "rush", "buzz". Just keep a note in a health diary to keep up your awareness of patterns at the root cause of triggers to uncover new ways of thinking. It may be easier to keep your diary entries in a light hearted doodling fashion.

The subject of what triggers any addiction cravings is very much a personal journey to uncover the root of the emotional needs that create a desire for an uplifted change in mood. This book is focusing more on physical addiction to chemicalism rather than the psychological and emotional triggers that drive any chemaholic.

Emotional triggers come from all directions with loss of love in a relationship or bereavement. There are many ways to handle the strong emotions with the support of helpful people.

There are many specialist charities offering telephone and face to face counselling. Seek out the specialist ones where possible for the better talking support. Talking therapy I recommend as it stands a chance of uncovering the truth long term. One alternative to feeling uncomfortable with some emotions is often a doctor's pill prescription to cover over the emotions short term. Having a healthy body is a good starting point to handling emotional stress triggers better and giving a sense of getting back control.

Each day I have a go at aiming for a balance of work, rest, play, and moderate exercise. With a little bit of food nutrition planning, I usually have a comfortable level of energy to do so. Very importantly, during every day, I aim to keep asking questions to learn more about nutrition and keep my awareness of what is triggering my appetite.

Summary

- Emotional stress and pleasure may trigger eating

- Solving one addiction may start another if the triggers are not overcome

- It is impossible to control people, places and things all the time

- Give disabled, vulnerable and sick people the best natural options available

- Seek out specialist talking therapy for long term serenity

STEP 8
Look younger by improved natural detoxing

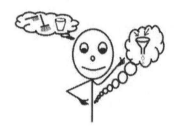

"The doctor of the future will no longer treat the human frame with drugs, but rather will cure and prevent disease with nutrition."

Thomas Edison

Inventor of the long lasting light bulb – movie camera & record player

"The more you eat, the less flavour, the less you eat, the more flavour."

Chinese Proverb

"Those who think they have no time for exercise will sooner or later have to find time for illness"

Edward Stanley

My 78 body organs have been put through a lot of physical stresses with a low nutrition lifestyle for over 30 years. I now decided to make amends to as many of my body organs as possible by detoxing them in a safe way, starting with the main organs.

This step may come across in a slightly different style than other steps. I feel it is important to highlight an awareness of the main organs and their detoxing functions of the body, emphasising the high percentages of water in them.

Through acupuncture treatments, I have understood better about how each body organ has a relationship with my emotions. I wanted to better the relationships between body organs and mind.

I had previously felt that some of my best organ (internal friends) had let me down in different ways. However, it was I who let them down. My thoughts, values, attitude were locked firmly into a chemaholic lifestyle. This caused my organs stress, which they in turn gave back to me. They were trying to help me by giving out many physical signals, aches, pains, inflammation, indigestion, and tinnitus. I was not listening to my body.

I am now thankful for any pains that previously were being heavily suppressed with a cocktail of painkillers. Now I listen for them, acknowledge their signals, and aim to respond better.

Severe feet pains forced me to get specialist hospital treatment in Wimbledon. The consultant explained I had Gout. The solution was a course of strong anti inflammatory drugs. Nausea and headaches were the main disabling side effects of the drugs making me so ill, unable to work.

These extreme side effects I reported on a yellow card. The card is sent to The government agency MHRA Medicines and Healthcare products Regulatory Agency regulates medicines. This helps build up data about medicines and in some cases after several years certain drugs have been withdrawn.

The real solution was a one month detox based on juicing fruits, homemade vegetable soup, no dairy products, no sweets or red wine. This was both a period of food deprivation and recovery. Once the pain had gone I went back to my previous habits and continued to increase my body weight.

Food goes in the mouth after being judged by sight, smell, and previous experiences. Touch and taste take over; provided the brain decides the food is acceptable it is chewed up (or swallowed). Enzymes from the mouth are chewed into the food to digest it and get it ready for swallowing. The secondary stage of digestion is in the stomach. I used to believe food was only digested in the stomach. Now I aim to chew up food properly so the stomach is not over worked, allowing the nutrition to be absorbed.

Treating each organ as a trusted valuable friend, I set about understanding what I had done to cause them harm, attempting amends without expectations or a quick fix. They needed to be convinced over several weeks that I was serious before they acknowledged my actions, rewarding me with feeling happier, having more youthful thinking and energy.

This involved making a list of them; anyone doing the same has to make their own list specific to them. I have found that lying quietly still and thinking about parts of my body is one way to tune into how different parts of my body are feeling.

Water makes up 50 -75% of the whole body, depending on the age and build of the person. However, the vital organs are made up of a higher percentage of water. It is essential to consume (99 % +) purified water when possible to help the best function of each organ. The percentage water is these organs are:

- Brain and spinal cord 73%
- Water and spleen 78%
- Lungs 83%
- Blood 83%

Spinal Cord 73% water

I put much stress on my body organs, and fortunately they did not fail enough to the point where I was close to death. However, I believe the cause of my lower spine area becoming highly inflamed was through Chemicalism. This resulted in acute, disabling, sciatic leg pain and years of chronic lower back pain. This was clear because, after many years of suffering with not being able to walk properly. I discovered that detoxing with homemade fresh vegetable soup took the inflammation down naturally. When the inflammation had gone down, the nerves and tissues were no longer under pressure. The spinal cord connects up the body, passing lots of messages to and from the brain. I believe with better nutrition and purified water, the mind functions better with improved signals.

Liver 71% water

It is a very robust organ from my experience. My doctor suggested 16 years ago I stop drinking high amounts of alcohol each day due to my blood tests confirming a very low (LFT) Liver Functioning Test. After I stopped consuming alcohol, my liver recovered enough to give back a normal blood test result within a few weeks because it still had the natural capacity to regenerate. This was fortunate as heavy alcoholics can damage their liver long term.

The liver is the largest internal organ with around 500 functions. It is the second most complex organ after the brain. Its functions include:

- Producing bile sending it to the stomach for digestion
- Filtering out toxins
- Regulating blood sugar
- Converts sugar, stores and releases it more

sugar is needed in the blood.

- Releasing cholesterol
- Breaking down fats
- Producing blood proteins
- Boosting immunity functions
- Regulating some hormones

It is like a busy factory with lots of workers in many departments reporting back to the brain every so often, but when the departments are treated badly with low wages / low nutrition, the factory starts to complain by working slowly or some departments going on strike!

Cancer Research uk.org shows one graph for UK, Males, 2010 -2012, with a 44% increase of deaths from liver cancer. This big increase suggests the very resilient liver organ is under an increasing strain to filter out toxins. I aim to help my liver keep up with its essential industrious work by drinking one organic fresh squeezed lemon in warm water most mornings. This provides the liver with extra detoxing respect. Usually I mix the lemon juice with Manuka honey.

Kidneys 79% water

Two kidneys filter water and salts out of the blood, producing urine. The kidneys produce an enzyme called rennin which regulates blood pressure. A healthy person is able to live with one kidney. The kidneys maintain the pH acidity and alkalinity levels of the blood. When I was obese eating mainly low nutrition food, this pattern would have tended to give me more of an acidic body and therefore more un-wellness.

Spleen 78% water

When I started on reducing my low nutrition lifestyle, my body started to naturally detox. I had a lot of body odour for a couple of weeks. Fortunately, I quickly read up on this to be reassured my body was working well. It is healthy to sweat out toxins.

The spleen is the largest organ in the lymphatic system, storing blood, filtering the blood, removing red blood cells with damage or over 120 days old that no longer carry oxygen effectively. Haemoglobin, the natural chemical carrying oxygen within the cells, gets broken down and recycled. The spleen plays a big role with fighting infection. Understanding this a bit more has helped me understand my blood tests which check for haemoglobin levels.

Stomach (Gut)

Food from the oesophagus goes to the stomach then to the small intestine. The stomach digests food by breaking it down, mixing it with digestive juices and enzymes.

Good instinctive emotional responses rather than considered thought come from the stomach (Gut), typical sayings being

"I had a gut feeling that something was wrong."

"I had a gut reaction."

I had previously assumed the body's intelligence came from the brain. Now my understanding of emotions coming from each organ has increased, particularly the gut. I have gained more useful intuition when my gut is giving me a sense of what feels good or bad when interpreting anything.

Small Intestine

Ninety percent of nutrients are absorbed in the small intestine digesting food using chemical enzymes. These nutrients go into the blood. The small intestine is incredibly long, over five meters. The food moves from the small intestine to the large intestine with muscle contractions and works. Eating four hours before sleeping gives the small intestine more of a chance to work better.

Muscles 79%

Muscles make up about 40 % of an average body weight with around 700 muscles in pairs. The busiest are around the eyes as they blink about 20,000 times a day and therefore require lubrication. Constant accumulation of acid in the body, through the lack of neutral PH water or low nutrition diet, makes muscles tired, tight and painful.

When I had acute sciatic pain, my acidity levels were high due to drinking mainly freshly squeezed oranges all the time as I believed this would help me get better through natural vitamin C. It was an allergy test that revealed the imbalance. I stopped drinking excessive amounts of orange juice and my pain reduced significantly with two weeks. A balance of acid and alkaline foods is essential for best health.

Bigger muscles burn up more calories.

Skin 64% water

This is the largest organ and has to maintain body temperature with sweat created to cool the body and goose bumps or raised hair to trap heat in the body. There are sweat and oil glands. The oil which the skin releases stops the skin from drying out or hair becoming brittle. Skin is able to absorb all kinds of chemicals, both nourishing and toxic.

Many types of creams, lotions, and facial makeup offer ways of improving younger looks and detoxing. Checking the ingredients of these products, just like food, is so important for giving the skin natural nutrition with natural minerals.

Natural ingredient shower and bath products from which the skin absorbs nutrition just like the body absorbs food need to be checked for their ingredients. For anyone with a skin complaint, this could be the source of a toxin, causing irritation. Having a relaxing bath with Himalayan bath salts absorbs natural trace minerals whilst detoxing the skin at the same time. There are many benefits of natural Himalayan bath salts, which have been a medicine for several thousand years.

Some people with sensitive skin get reactions from washing up liquid, so it is possible to buy natural washing up liquid at a similar price to avoid the cause. I found that cooking natural foods somehow does not require me to use washing up liquid very much. Nowadays I mainly use hot water only, just spending extra time cleaning. The other benefit of using just hot water is the washing up liquid no longer features in the daily intake of artificial chemicals. Without washing up liquid used to clean the cups, I find tea tastes better and has no bubbles.

Blood 83%

Normal, natural blood pressure maybe gained through consuming high nutrition, taking some exercise regularly and handling every day stress calmly with humility when possible. Blood is the fluid delivering essential oxygen, nutrients, sugar and hormones throughout the body. Blood also collects waste from cells to be flushed out the body in urine, faeces, sweat, and exhaled through the lungs. High quality purified water is our life blood.

Colon, Rectum, Anus

From the stomach, digested foods pass through two parts of the intestines, firstly the colon, then the rectum, with the final waste leaving the body through the anus.

The colon absorbs water; when absorption is low, there is diarrhoea; when absorption is high, there is constipation. Constipation provides a fertile breeding area for toxic waste to be reintroduced back into the body through the blood stream.

Regular passing of waste is essential for natural body detoxing. The colon needs to be functioning smoothly to prevent many known diseases and provide a high quality of life.

I believe the colon, like the gut, has an emotional

effect on the whole body. The first time someone has a colonic irrigation, they normally are surprised by an immediate feeling of well-being and energy.

The colour of healthy faeces is light brown with smooth texture. Unhealthy faeces are hard, cobbled and very dark brown or black looking. Unhealthy digestion brings with it bad odours from flatulence and when going to the toilet, bad odour. These are all signs the body is helpfully giving out and which have a direct relationship to nutrition.

Living in a world with lots of toxins

Modern day popular illnesses such as obesity, cancer and mental illnesses are on the increase are partly due to people living longer. Many people, including scientists who have authored published research studies, clearly understand the causes. It is not always possible to promote all the solutions due to overwhelming logistical, commercial or funding implications.

It took many years before medical data proved smoking was an unhealthy lifestyle option.

When I gave up smoking the next best alternative has been burning frankincense. There are many different types with various calming or uplifting qualities. More easily available are incense sticks which can also assist when giving up smoking.

The chances of giving up smoking increases by having a new lifestyle plan involving support. Talking through the options with a doctor, pharmacy and hypnotherapist are all good starting points. I was helped by a book Allen Carr's Easy Way To Stop Smoking.

The only real way forward is for individuals (and carers of individuals) is to take personal responsibility for detoxing each day as best as possible. This maintains a tolerable level of toxins absorbed and processed in the body.

The many clever body organs are designed to handle a level of filtering or detoxing while absorbing nutrition. Being aware of their water percentage content emphasis the need to give them each (neutral ph) purified water.

There is much pollution in the world and artificial chemicals to be aware of in the food chain. Regular personal detoxing using purified water and sufficiently high nutrition food are essential for enjoying a healthy lifestyle.

Consuming all high nutrition food and drinks that require no detoxing is probably only possible in a laboratory environment.

There is so much to know about each of the physical parts of the body, so take a very simple approach. Focusing on detoxing your body with:

- Purified (99%) water supply

- Long enough rested sleep

- Natural high nutrition 80% to cope with 20% low nutrition

I believe a healthy workable lifestyle is to aim for consuming a high level of natural nutrition to strengthen the body's natural detoxing ability, keeping immunity high. This helps avoid much un-wellness, minimising medicinal drugs. Also, very importantly, the body is able to consume and or enjoy low nutrition favourite choices of food and drink without feeling deprived.

Summary

- The body is mostly water 50 -75% depending on age and build

- Body organs contain up to 79% water

- Blood uses the highest percentage of water 83%

- It is essential to consume quality water with minimal toxins

STEP 9

Enjoy a new level of better health

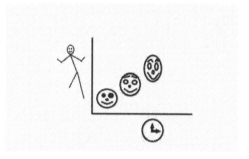

"Healing is a matter of time, but it is sometimes also a matter of opportunity."

Hippocrates, Greek Philosopher

"The part can never be well unless the whole is well."

Plato, Greek Philosopher

It was a busy time as a suffering chemaholic with a list of illnesses that dominated my lifestyle, especially the obesity with the mental torment about food options.

Chronic pains in my lower back, acute sciatic leg pains, and aching shoulders kept me busy with medical visits squashed into a busy working life. Now, with a new healthier lifestyle, I appreciate having more time to look deeper into enjoying better health.

Some of the solutions for better natural health may not fall into conventional, well-known categories, so I attempt to keep an open mind about the limitless number of natural health solutions, however they present themselves.

I understand successfully going from failure to failure without loss of enthusiasm (as Winston Churchill said) and searching for a health remedy require an increasing determination with moments of doubt. I urge anyone with any illness to keep an open mind and to continue searching among the thousands of established, proven, natural remedies.

Someone may say to me "I have tried every possible remedy available." I know this is ONLY BELIEF and NOT FACT. Only if they had consulted in some way with leading experts on natural health in each of the 196 countries, read extensively about historic remedies, be up to date with the latest technological and scientific advancements would I accept that all possibilities have been considered. I would feel that way until tomorrow because new health solutions are being discovered and rediscovered every day!

Assertively avoid being trapped into a dead end corner by the beliefs of any other person or organisation who wants to convince you that there are no solutions to a health problem.

Become highly aware of prescribed drug side effects from the drug manufacturers information so it is clear what can be expected.

Alternative Medicine and treatments

They are in limitless supply. I have benefited a lot from many of the most established, easily available, alternative treatments including:

- Acupuncture,
- Aromatherapy
- Reflexology
- Homeopathy
- Osteopathy
- Chiropractic methods
- Cupping
- Reflexology
- Hydrotherapy

Natural remedies aim to cure the source normally without side effects. They may work more slowly or quickly than prescribed drug treatments.

Homeopathy is one of the more controversial alternative medicines since it was invented in 1796. Homeopathy has cured me and many of my friends from unusual incurable illnesses. It works much like an inoculation by giving the person a small dose of the illness. However, scientific research says it only works like a placebo. If that is the truth, then my friends and I are glad to respond well to placebos.

Once my own main un-wellness of obesity had gone it was time to solve other long term health issues. By getting rid of long term health problems I started to feel much younger.

Mouth - Dentistry and Taste

After two years of multiple tooth aches for which five dentists; aided by X-rays and one hospital consultant; could not locate the source, I was fed up with suffering.

When I was in Poland in 2014, a university professor, Ala, used some advanced natural healing techniques on me which immediately pinpointed a deep jaw infection. On my return to the UK, I had it treated by two brilliant private dentists. They reluctantly drilled into what appeared on X-rays as a healthy tooth. They were surprised to discover an unusually big, trapped infection that took three treatments during a week to release.

I did take prescribed antibiotics to kill bacteria. I knew the antibiotics kill both bad and good bacteria; I also took extra probiotics to regenerate good bacteria for digestion.

Getting my teeth fixed up meant I was able to chew and crunch food without pain or uncomfortable aching.

Chewing my food longer allows many natural enzymes produced in the mouth to start breaking down the food immediately and also improves flavour. After consuming high nutrition, organic food for about six to eight weeks, my taste buds went through the roof. It is a real joy to have all my own teeth in good condition. Now I have no aches or pains, able to chew and crunch so that the digestion process is working better.

De-clutter the mind

One part of my health I had overlooked for many years was being mildly cluttered. My eyes told me so, and it had been tiring. I did not know it until after a big spring clean. The more I de-cluttered the more layers of clutter I found from keys on a key ring, old mobile phones boxes and bags.

Now I was enjoying the successful results of spring cleaning my kitchen cupboards. It made spring cleaning other areas of my new lifestyle fun, using my new mindset, not being afraid to throw away or give away redundant items. My eyes told my mind to feel clearer. The more de-cluttering I completed, the more hidden things appeared, some useful. I gained extra space but more importantly a big sense of freedom through improved mental clarity.

There is an addiction that involves a compulsion to gather and clutter to the point of suffering. There is an organisation that has developed a 12 step recovery program of recovery.

My book shelves full of many health books needed a sort out to see what would be immediately useful. It was about going from *shelf development* to *self-development*. Many books were no longer required, so they went to the charity shops. I rediscovered many good books to read. For example, I no longer required a book on how to cure tinnitus (ringing in the ears) because I no longer suffered from it due to my high nutrition diet. Finding useful books and paperwork more easily is a new subtle pleasure for a happier lifestyle.

It is amazing how much clutter I had accumulated, especially boxes, bags and containers. Clearing a whole attic over many weeks created a new usable room that was my reward. The same thought process took place when I cleared out the low nutrition foods from the kitchen cupboards. The benefits of clearing old clutter or unwanted belongings have given me unexpected mental freedom. I believe this has helped my overall health with extra calm. My eyes confirmed to my mind I had a more organised new lifestyle. It is a good feeling to find things quickly.

Regular exercise

This has been a good healer for me because of increased circulation. Any moderate exercise every day is good, however small. Making new goals for exercise is now fun. Just visiting a leisure centre for a sauna and Jacuzzi all counts towards an uplifting healthy lifestyle. The natural foods help increase oxygen flowing around the body, which aids healing. With my body having changed from an unhealthy acidic level to an alkaline one, I naturally have more energy. Regular movement tones muscle strength.

Q10 Coenzyme

The body naturally produces coenzyme Q10. This coenzyme is available over the counter in pharmacists and health stores as a supplement. Q10 helps cells produce energy, acting as an antioxidant that improves immunity. Q10 is very good for increasing natural energy levels after about thirty days.

Timing of enjoying new levels of better health

These 12 steps make up a basic plan to support a lifestyle change over several months, moving from un-wellness and obesity to enjoyable improved health. There is no time limit on each step because everyone has their own pace; the main thing is to continue while enjoying improvements.

Peeling away more layers of un-wellness with new solutions along the way has encouraged me to listen, hear, and respond better to the natural signals of my body.

Treat yourself for making good progress with your improved health!

Food combinations

By combining the right food types this improves digestion. Being slim is generally associated with being young. To lose weight naturally I sensed a revived feeling of youthfulness. To start tuning the body better with food combinations tunes up the digestive system to the next level. This is not covered in this book because it needs to be explained in detail to make sense of food combinations and there are many books dedicated to this one subject.

Summary

- Look for natural remedies and treatments to get rid of long term un-wellness

- There is a big supply of natural remedies from all around the world

- Teeth are important for enjoying food and digestion

- De-clutter generally and gain a new level of freedom with extra space to see

- Food combinations there is lots to find out

STEP 10
Review and adjust

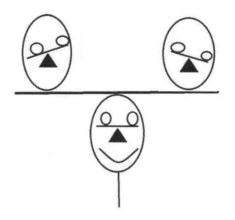

"Intelligence is the ability to adapt to change."
Stephen Hawking - physicist, cosmologist, author

"When antibiotics first came out, nobody could have imagined we'd have the resistance problem we face today. We didn't give bacteria credit for being able to change and adapt so fast."
Bonnie Bassler - Professor in Molecular Biology

"Your mind is the most powerful medicine."
Louise Hay – self healed from cancer – writer

Ongoing success requires some regular reviewing and plan adjusting. It is easier to stay well than get well.

Having made so many lifestyle changes gradually. I saw better results in my blood tests every few weeks. This factual feedback is so encouraging. The blood tests after six months showed significant improvements with cholesterol and glucose down to normal.

My ITIL qualification in I.T. impressed upon me that quality changes involve an ongoing review to keep things working well based on a measured feedback. I have full blood tests done every six months.

New nutrition attitude

The most important review after several months is to acknowledge how new beliefs about food have allowed a person to say goodbye to many symptoms. Review the twelve common symptoms of a chemaholic listed in chapter one after the front index.

Automatically checking the source of food all the time has become normal, and now it is easy to spot low nutrition, chemaholic products marketed with healthy sounding phases. Nutrition checking has replaced just price comparison. It is a more interesting new game with the reward of better health to enjoy.

How healthy are you?

With good health and improving health, expect a false sense of security. As layers of illness and then better health are revealed, it is wise to keep aware with tests about the facts. It is fair to say health can always be improved, and people are always so surprised when a healthy looking person suddenly passes away.

More ideas for recovering chemaholics

- Thirty meals in thirty days was a first challenge. Has this become a new habit? How about introducing more organic, gluten free products into a high nutrition lifestyle for snacks and desserts and have a party or celebration with friends?

- Have one day a week of organic and natural nutrition only.

- Visit a show that is dedicated to organic, vegan or natural foods.

- The 100 challenge. Now that you have practiced digesting food in the mouth by chewing food thoroughly and gaining extra taste before swallowing, is it now possible to eat a full mouthful of food and chew 100 hundred times before swallowing? Yes. This process brings extra taste and satisfies a chewing hunger which the brain uses to judge when appetite has been satisfied. I can easily get over 100 chews with a mouthful of toasted organic rye bread.

- Hands free. Is it possible to eat a sandwich and put it down in between mouthfuls until each mouthful is digested with chewing and swallowed? Yes. Holding food whilst eating speeds up eating food, so experiments suggest slowing down will lead to higher enjoyment.

- Nutrition is king. Is it possible to buy a chemaholic style meal or expensive snack, enjoy the first few mouthfuls while fully chewing and digesting, and be satisfied enough with the initial flavour? Re-judge. If you decide it is not good enough quality, discard the rest because it no longer is tasty even though it has been paid for.

- Be in a group of chemaholics and choose natural food options and fully digest with chewing, not conforming to group pressure.

- Eat before or without alcohol so the alcohol does not affect appetite judgment, usually leading to less of an appetite for food and alcohol.

- Being aware of the sources of non-chemically produced genetically modified vegetables, uncover new local sources of low cost organic vegetables or home grown. Growing vegetables and fishing can be a free source of high nutrition and a money saving option.

- Preference for natural food tastes has become so strong because the natural taste far exceeds the chemical versions of the same foods. Have a go at returning to low nutrition food for a few days. Notice any increased tiredness, weight changes, and any other unwanted symptoms so you are more confident with food options. If there is weight gain or unwanted symptoms, make a note of how long it takes to return to normal. There is no need to feel guilty so take it easy.

Tests

There are so many tests available due to the advancement of technology and medical techniques. Home testing is much easier with many medical stores selling self-testing machines or kits for blood pressure, glucose, allergies. Cancer tests and risk assessment using DNA offer a wide range of options especially privately. There are specially trained dogs able to detect cancers in humans using their highly sensitive smell.

Eyesight, hearing, fitness tests and whatever other tests are easily available to help work out how to improve quality of life, adjusting and treating. I discovered my tinnitus (continuous ringing in the ears) had virtually disappeared to the point I had forgotten about it, all thanks to the dietary changes.

Nerve feeling sensations came back in my lower right leg in 2013. These feelings I was told would never return due to a severed nerve below my knee in a motorbike accident in 2011. I was lucky to get to first aid within minutes of the accident as I had a severed artery with blood pumping out. Acupuncture has been done regularly to re grow the nerve. The test on my leg to check the nerve signal was done in a hospital with an electrical current measurement. It was painful but it was good to know the signal was getting through.

Keep testing and keep a note in your health diary.

Food intolerance and allergy

Allergies may be life threatening, so a medical approach through a doctor is best. Most people describe food intolerances as allergies.

The test results for intolerances may show up more accurate results after consuming mainly high nutrition for at least two months, incorporating probiotic foods or probiotic supplements to strengthen immunity. Probiotics are used to restore the natural balance of essential gut bacteria.

Knowing about your food intolerances, avoiding them, or building up stronger tolerance can bring about an improved quality of life.

Food intolerances and allergies have increased a lot in recent years. This has caused a mini commercial boom with gluten free and "frees from" products. European legislation introduced in 2005 makes food producers' state allergy warnings on the packaging.

I often wonder if some chemaholic foods cause an inflammation in the stomach which is mistaken for a temporary feeling of fullness.

Cancer

There are many types of cancers. Cancer Research UK states a healthy diet can reduce the risk of cancer.

My experience of being diagnosed with cancer by The NHS was a big shock in 2008. I went to work the next day in a daze and started to think about how to tidy up my life's affairs so they were all in order for my loved ones. I found much compassion from other people who had also handled the shock of being diagnosed with cancer. However, nobody told me about the possible cures available through diet.

Fortunately, I do not have cancer. I am now very interested in the importance of having high immunity through good nutrition and purified water.

The body generates new cells everyday, automatically self-destroying the bad or old ones through strong immunity systems.

To contribute to someone else's life indirectly, donating healthy blood always feels good. It also provides a personal health check.

Cancer is often considered a modern day health condition because of the growing number of detected and treated cases every year.

Cancer Research UK website accessed May 2016

Provides an explanation with graph about why more people get cancer.

http://scienceblog.cancerresearchuk.org/2015/02/04/why-are-cancer-rates-increasing/

Growing problem

By far the biggest risk factor for most cancers is simply getting older. More than three-quarters of all people diagnosed with cancer in the UK are over the age of 60.

And this is because cancer is a disease of our genes – the bits of DNA code that hold the instructions for all of the microscopic machinery inside our cells. Over time, mistakes accumulate in this code – scientists can now see them stamped in cancer's DNA. And it's these mistakes that can kick start a cell's journey towards becoming cancerous.

The longer we live, the more time we have for errors to build up. And so, as time passes, our risk of developing cancer goes up, as we accumulate more of these faults in our genes.

In the graph below, you can see how UK life expectancy has increased over time and the number of people living into old age is higher than ever before.

This means there are now more people than ever living to an age where they have a higher risk of developing cancer.

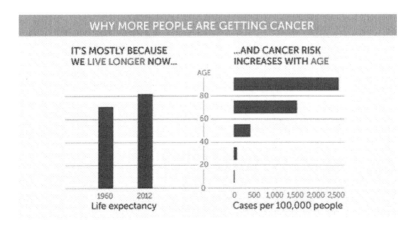

But we **can** stack the odds of avoiding cancer in our favour. Things that happen throughout our lives can speed up – or slow down – the rate at which errors occur in our genes. These include things we can control, and some we can't.

They include our lifestyle, our genetics & family history, our exposure to viruses, the job we do, the air we breathe – and they can all play different roles in our overall risk of developing the disease.

Thank you to www.cancerresearchuk.org for allowing the reproduction of the above graph and explanation.

We create cancer cells every day; it is up to a healthy immune system to kill the cancer cells, stopping them from multiplying.

The older a person becomes the higher odds of a lower immunity, therefore a higher chance of getting cancer.

The U.K Cancer Research Organisation explains in their lifestyle information that cancer risks are reduced by eating less processed foods.

The responsibility is clearly upon the individual to get tested as preventative.

If the government health service detects cancer at any stage, they can only do their best to cure the condition. Prevention is the best cure, and to keep blood as alkaline as possible, by eating natural food options.

Professor Jane Plant explains in her book "Beat Cancer," how she healed her cancer by diet.

After spending several weeks putting into practice steps one to nine, have a look at step one, "Common Symptoms of a Chemaholic." You may have been suffering from all twelve symptoms. Just for fun, how about give one point to each symptom from which you are now suffering. This process may give you an indication of how well things are going with your healthier, everyday, natural, detoxing lifestyle.

Summary

- Chewing more improves flavour and digestion

- Food allergy and intolerances be sure what they are and which ones have gone

- Cancer is more common as an illness and more curing exists

- Always remember step one

STEP 11
Resting detox
and peaceful balance

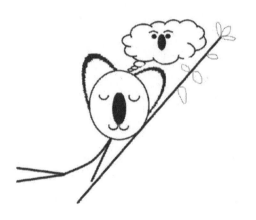

"If you can't sleep, then get up and do something instead of lying there worrying. It's the worry that gets you, not the lack of sleep."
Dale Carnegie

"Two things define you: Your patients when you have nothing, and your attitude when you have everything"
Just an inspiring tweet@Lolly Daskal May 2016
Coach Speaker Author

We spend around 25 years sleeping in an average lifetime. With quality sleep, life expectancy is increased.

The Australian Koala (often known as koala bear) is the longest sleeping mammal, up to 22 hours per day. (Human beings are mammals.) Koalas live on nutrition from eucalyptus tree leaves which is:

- Very low nutrition
- Highly toxic
- High fibre diet
- Difficult-to-digest

As they have a low nutrition diet, they have low energy. Sleeping is their essential way of surviving and conserving energy. The gum trees have leaves that are highly toxic to stop insects eating them. The koala has developed a natural way to detoxify the leaves through slow digestion. They also have a slow metabolic rate, whilst extracting the maximum nutrition.

Detoxing through the right amount of sleep is essential for high immunity. Human brain cells reduce by around 60% when asleep. This allows the glymphatic system to work ten times harder than awake to clear out brain specific toxins built up whilst awake.

I imagine this brain detox process much like Disney World: busy during the day and host to large crowds of thrill-seeking people who all go home to sleep at night. Then the night-time cleaning staffs are able to rush around ten times faster without the visiting crowds; making it easier to clean up all the areas; fix broken bits, and take away the previous day's rubbish to be ready for the next day's business.

Lack of sleep

Headaches, loss of memory, difficulty solving problems, nausea, lack of coordination, tiredness, and increased appetite are common signs of sleep deprivation. These symptoms are easy for most people to fix temporarily using over the counter drugs and caffeine drinks.

Sleep deprivation is a well known successful form of torture used in wartimes. There are many elite military training regiments that include overcoming this torture technique such as The Royal Marine Commandos.

The metabolism works best when a person gets good sleep every day, helping maintain an ideal body weight through hormones. With lack of sleep, two hormones, leptin and ghrelin, become unbalanced, leading to increased hunger and weight gain.

Blood pressure also gets high with lack of sleep.

Bed

From my experience, the best type of bed needs a mattress and pillow that feels very comfortable. There are many options, including memory foam products which continually mould into the body when asleep. Whilst I had several years of not able to walk properly, I have always stuck with a 1000 pocket sprung mattress. Nowadays I am lucky enough to also enjoy camping and take a self inflating back roll to support my lower back.

Light

Sleeping without light is the best way for maximum quality sleep. Consider blackout curtains or blinds. Keep doors closed that allow light in. Clocks and electrical items that glow or have lights can be moved around to avoid disturbance. I use a purposefully made blindfold when sleeping in the daytime, on a plane, or just sleeping somewhere that has a lot of light.

Having a jug of purified water by the bedside is helpful whenever waking up thirsty in the middle of a sleep period. That way, you avoid turning on lights and waking up the brain with activities that prolong disturbed sleep.

Noise

Noise disturbs sleep it is a valuable survival instinct. Aim for a quiet place to rest when possible. When I was sleeping in my flat in 2009 a fire broke out below in the shop after they had closed. The fumes from the fire had sent me into a deep sleep. People woke me up by banging on the first floor double glazed window before the fire engines arrived. The noise woke me up before the smoke (carbon monoxide poisoning) killed me. Fortunately after coming back from the hospital I suffered no illness.

Breathing

Air in the home can often need cleaning up. On long haul flights the aeroplanes have HEPA air filters which clean up the recycled cabin air. It is possible to buy domestic HEPA air filters in many sizes which look like a fan. The HEPA filter takes out 85–99.9 % of particles floating in the air. These filters are very good to help sleeping for asthma and hay fever sufferers or people who need maximum quality air at night time.

My cat fluffy had a permanent summertime skin irritation which recovered due to having a HEPA filter cleaning the air for a few hours every day. This saved money on vet's bills for steroid injections that were no longer required.

When I was obese it was difficult to get a good sleep having been diagnosed with sleep apnea. I had an operation on the inside of my nose cutting away the bone to increase my airways.

Temperature

Core body temperature drops when asleep, so it is good to be cool when sleeping and approaching the sleep period. After coming out of a hot bath or sauna, the body automatically starts working on cooling down in preparation for sleep. I often have a sauna two hours before sleeping to both clear the skin of toxins from the day and enhance sleep.

Many of our basic survival instincts come from the need to stay alive. The dark of night provides safety and a cooler temperature to rest.

Feet

Foot detox pads maybe a gimmick; however, I use them occasionally as has my mum, who recovered from terminal feet gangrene in 2014. Many friends have agreed they ease aching feet.

Smell

Essential oils help me get to sleep; the best one recommended to me many years ago is clary sage, or if not easily available, lavender.

Digestion rest time

Eating close to sleep is often due to habits rather than necessity, so with a bit of planning, a new lifestyle can bring new habits with new late night natural snacks. Giving the body a rest from digestion allows it to recover. Consuming foods with sugar or caffeine before sleeping keeps the brain awake.

After a good sleep, I follow the proven way of starting up my digestive system with fresh organic lemon juice in warm purified water. I understand this increases immunity with anti-bacterial and antiviral properties. Weight loss improves through better digestion and cleaning the liver.

Lemons, although acidic, once inside the body, alkalise. This helps keep the blood in a natural alkaline state, absorbing more oxygen. Disease occurs when the blood moves towards an acid state. Many low nutrition foods impact upon the blood by increasing the acidity, so drinking fresh organic lemon juice in water is my daily antidote for maintaining an alkaline blood PH level. (This is not the same as stomach acid).

The better immunity achieved through good quality sleep means less illness and more time to get on with life.

Meditation

There are many different styles of meditation. It has been proven to lower blood pressure. Most people know it is practiced for relaxation, overcoming anxiety and depression. I aim to grab 20 minutes a day as "my time" to escape into selfish relaxation. I recommend this to anyone wanting to calm down from a busy workaholic lifestyle.

Meditation and power napping for many people have been alternatives to sleep at night or day. All rest is good when it is difficult to get the full number of hours for quality sleep. Short meditations have many benefits for improved well-ness.

Being in a peaceful and still position with an open mind is associated with connecting to a higher spiritual power. There is no reference to God in this book. Everyone has an understanding of their own helpful higher power.

Hypnosis has worked for me in many ways to access to my subconscious with hypnosis CDs. There are many internet downloads and videos available which are playable on a smart phone.

Spiritual

International healer and speaker Shirley Rhodes uses her many sayings to describe spiritual happiness which are:

* We can find the answers within us but never be afraid to ask for help and support always

* Spiritual is anything, it's all encompassing good energy

* Coincidental happenings can be helpful

* Your body is your temple

* Be open to signs on your journey

* Have "your time" short rest periods to become unavailable, switch off technology and close the door

* Each person is special

* The way we think can take us towards addictions

- Learn with baby steps
- Find answers inside yourself to feel calmer

It's a challenge every 24 hours

Sleep detoxing is one of the most challenging parts of my lifestyle. A small amount of preparation each night is a good investment for the next day's mental ability. I empathise with anyone who is working to improve their detoxing sleep because it is so essential for a balanced, happy lifestyle with energy. There are so many factors that reduce good sleep such as stress. Being prepared with proven ways to increase a good sleep is good enough as life is not perfect.

Summary

- Sleep allows detoxing for the brain
- Avoid sleep deprivation torture
- Weight loss or maintaining a healthy body is helped with deep sleep
- Light and noises disturb sleep
- Meditation is calming and aids digestion
- Spiritual happiness
- Rest is good for reducing stress and increases immunity

STEP 12

Passing on your enriched lifestyle in order to attract more well-being

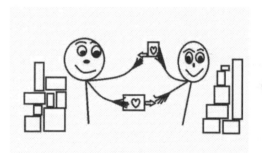

What you give out is what you get back

"No act of kindness, however small, is ever wasted."

Aesop writer of fables

"You can have everything in life you want, if you will just help other people get what they want."

Zig Ziglar author and motivational speaker

*"To know even one life has breathed easier because
you have lived. This is to have succeeded."*

Ralph Waldo Emerson, poet and philosopher

"Service to others is the rent you pay for your room here on earth."

Muhammad Ali world champion boxer

"You can take a horse to the water but you cannot make it drink."

Proverb

About two months into this plan, I gave up feeling fear towards food as I had accepted that real high nutrition natural food is to be loved, not feared.

Initially, I had to move out of my rigid mental comfort zone, swapping what I had believed for years were the healthiest slimming options. This new approach gradually changed something every few days to build up my confidence with natural food and drinks.

My body adjusted without any major objections, avoiding major cravings.

It does take courage to let go of strongly held beliefs just a day at a time. I had slight weight gain at times, so I decided to only weigh myself once a week and keep my thoughts focused on enjoying higher nutrition foods as the number one priority plus regular moderate exercise.

Once I started to feel better than I had for years, thoughts about a return to the old lifestyle were easy to dismiss.

It took a big leap of faith for me to believe just eating mainly natural organic foods and drinking purified water with regular moderate exercise would give me a whole new enjoyable lifestyle. Now that I am convinced about chemicalism. I want to share this with everyone interested who wants to spoil themselves with good health from eating fewer chemicals and more natural nutrition.

For many people, sharing the benefits and joy of natural nutrition extends to their animal friends, pets, cats and dogs. There are now natural vitamin and mineral supplements for pets. Perhaps one day the ingredients of tinned pet food may become more regulated regarding the ingredients. My cat Fluffy had his favourite natural foods such as prawns. I was always amazed at his unusually extra fast consumption of a portion of certain expensive, processed cat treats. There was something in them that gave him a ravenous appetite more than any type of natural foods. Healthier nutrition for pets and animals may also save on the vet's bills.

Knowing my chemaholic limits to building Confidence

By comparison, people who like to drink alcohol usually get to know their limits on how much to consume: how long and how often, the side effects from multiple experiences, and the short term recovery time. It is helpful to know what to expect about the recovery periods so it is easier to make better decisions for a happier lifestyle.

Bounce Back Test One

After about four months, I tested out my resilience when consuming toxic and low nutrition foods and drinks. I was interested mainly in relation to weight gain and loss rates to know more about the natural response of how long it would take to recover.

In one day I consumed three big chemaholic meals with lots of snacks, which kept me feeling very bloated throughout the day. I was treating it as a fun test, and it reminded me what life used to be like as normal. It was good aversion therapy.

Also I ate fast, gulping to minimise digestion, drank alcohol, and made sure everything I consumed had maximum sugar. After a few drinks, later in the evening, my appetite became confusingly stimulated. This helped me to keep awake and eat lots of sweet snacks I had specially bought in. I fell asleep by accident watching TV, waking up in the middle of the night and remembering I was doing this crazy test.

The next day I had low energy for a few hours after waking and felt constipated, so I bought some natural laxatives. The unpleasant smells I created when using the toilet reminded me what life used to be like as a suffering chemaholic with regular indigestion.

The unpleasant wind–flatulence throughout the day made me feel embarrassed around others. Also later in the day, I bought an air freshener spray for the toilet, again another added expense of my previous chemaholic lifestyle.

I had no noticeable weight gain or loss that day, so I concluded my body could recover from the side effects of a full-on over-the-top chemaholic binge within a day.

My one day test was very full-on.

Bounce back test two

I ate only low nutrition food for three days just like I used to but which no longer had much appeal. The chemaholic food had less and less flavour, and my taste buds were craving tasty organic foods. Energy and enthusiasm went down, but I knew it was worth sticking with this test to get to know how long I could last for before my weight started to increase. Unlike the first test, this was much more moderate. I planned it for one week, so I stocked up with a load of low cost, chemaholic processed meals, foods, and drinks.

After three days, I started to gain weight. I was fed up with the tiredness, so my one week experiment was cut short to just three days. I did this three day experiment several times with a similar result each time. The process reinforced my pleasure in tasting high nutrition meals and snacks. The good news is that after one week of returning to normal, natural foods, my weight and feeling of wellbeing had returned to normal.

I was also very pleased that without any hesitation I was able to throw away all the chemaholic meals and foods very happily, as they had no real value to me anymore.

Bounce back test three - warning

This one week test of consuming chemaholic foods happened by accident and was not planned when I was on holiday in Malta. Fortunately, I had a lot of time in the day to reflect on my holiday eating habits, realising how quickly I had become addicted back to a chemaholic diet.

I consumed low nutrition food over seven days on meals included with the holiday which made me feel unwell and very tired. After returning to my normal 80 % natural nutrition lifestyle, I found that it took around three to four weeks for my body to naturally resettle back to my normal weight with energy.

This is very reassuring to know and has taken away a certain fear about what happens when suddenly the majority of nutrition is not natural, which can happen for all kinds of unexpected reasons. If you are planning to challenge yourself with this kind of test, you need to be very careful because it can be extremely dangerous to your health. Therefore, my legal friend told me I cannot recommend any dangerous test. Keep these (as I call them) bounce back tests moderate with natural nutrition available as a food first aid if possible. Once a living body of any person, animal, insect is working well with high natural nutrition then receives a high amount of poisonous toxins, the change is highly likely to cause noticeable illness or even death in some cases. This has been shown in the study of the declining population of bee colonies due to pesticide toxicity.

This one week unplanned test made me hit upon and strengthen a new level of understanding about how easy it is to become mentally re-addicted to artificial chemicals in food and drink. Also I aim for detoxing holidays nowadays!

Nutrition Feasting Test

Natural, high nutrition foods burn off quickly. I experimented eating large amounts of high nutrition foods to see how many days it would take to increase weight. It seemed the more high nutrition foods I consumed, the more energy I had to burn off with exercise rather than put weight on. After seven athletic days, I had put on no noticeable extra weight and had enjoyed lots of extra cycling.

One Sunday lunchtime during my week of high nutrition feasting test. I went for a casual cycle ride which was planned to last for two hours with an ambitious distance of potentially 40 kilometres to Boxhill in Surrey. It was a sunny day. However, with so much unexpected energy, I enthusiastically enjoyed carrying on, cycling from London to the seaside town of Worthing. This journey covered around 110 kilometres in six hours. The last time I had cycled this far, I was aged 15 years!

When coming home by train the same day, I did experience some painful leg cramps. After this long cycle ride, I ended this week of testing myself as my muscles and overall body were suffering from over-exercising. Also, my solo adventure was at the cost of missing meeting up with some good friends. A few days later, my leg muscles had become much stronger when cycling. I concluded it is important to keep a balance of high nutrition foods and some exercise, avoiding getting addicted in a suffering way to the natural high of over-exercising.

These tests are not for everyone, and everybody is different. In my mum's case (aged 93 years), during one week she went from having very stiff aching arthritic hands to having full function in all fingers, no pain, and proud to be in charge of chopping all the household organic vegetables.

Holding onto these moments of good healthy achievement I feel is very important. I had taken a selfie next to the sign to Worthing sign with my cycle also I took photos and a video of my mum chopping up vegetables. Looking back on these photos can be very therapeutic and inspiring, especially when the pictures bring a healthy smile.

It is a good idea to get to know again your new physical health limits, becoming more attuned to your body's abilities. Testing yourself with a little extra exercise at your own pace is one way to build or rebuild an improved level of confidence. Very moderate exercise can take place right now for 30 seconds! Before doing any ambitious exercise, give yourself a fair chance of enjoyable success with some preparation, picking a good time such as a day off of work or avoiding days of menstruation to make steady progress. Knowing physical limits is also potentially life-saving. The main thing is to know yourself.

Most of all, have fun learning that your new lifestyle changes have rewarded you with better health and a more confident self.

Trusting in myself has increased by testing how my body reacts to chemicalism.

People like to discuss how they are confused about food

I recommend passing on information about Chemicalism to other open minded people, as it is very rewarding to see people become happier as they change their lifestyles for the better. It also builds a support group.

Premature death from illness can be very motivating for a person to have an open mind for change. I always aim to spend more time explaining about Chemicalism to people who believe they are suffering chemaholics and want to take immediate action.

After reducing in weight by 22 kilos in six months, gradually people I had not seen for a while asked me what had happened.

At first I was excited to tell anyone who would listen about how I was losing weight, getting fitter. Elsa explained that over many years people often asked her how she stays younger looking with above average health. However, because the easy answers she gives usually threaten a person's beliefs too much, only a few people have listened to her excellent advice from which I have much more to learn.

Many people told me they had expected to hear I had become unwell through cancer, discovered a magic pill, gotten on a new gimmick diet, or gotten committed to working out at a gym. When I explained with enthusiasm how changing to natural food options produced an improved healthy lifestyle, conversations soon ended. I realised most people feel more comfortable discussing many ways of not succeeding with their frustrating beliefs because it is easier to relate to.

The easiest explanation I have used is "I have changed to mainly organic and gluten free foods avoiding artificial chemicals when possible."

People want a quick answers from reliable sources they trust.

When someone explains to me they eat healthily with lots of fresh vegetables, I ask did they used to eat non fresh vegetables. Do they choose the ones sprayed with pesticides or organic? Do they wash and boil them with 99% purified water or use tap water containing weed killer? If these answers offend someone's beliefs too much, I refrain. Only offering extra explanations if asked and hope they may follow up on these ideas with their own research.

When someone explains to me they drink lots of water to detox I ask whether the water comes with weed killer from the tap or is it 99% purified water. If it is bottled water they use, I ask if they like to choose spring water, natural mineral water, or the normal low cost bottled water. These three types of water are regulated by U.K. E.U. legislation. "Bottled water" is tap water put into a container that does not say "spring" or "natural mineral water" and legally is sold in shops.

Chemaholics with little awareness of tasty natural foods are locked into their own fear of "how will I cope with life without tasty chemaholic food fixes?" It is only by taking action, tasting the natural alternatives and finding the flavours to be enjoyed more than imagined that this fear can be easily overcome or reduced in steps.

It is not always possible to go about a normal working, social life without consuming a percentage of artificial, chemically processed food and drinks each week, so I aim to keep it low when possible. "Take it easy." Simple planning helps a lot whilst enjoying the freedom of eating without fear.

Often one addiction is removed, another and another will appear. My first addiction of being a workaholic had the same outward side an effect of other addictions. Addiction is about seeking a "fix" to be happy. It maybe to escape from uncomfortable emotions. I keep on the lookout in my lifestyle to aim for a balance of being aware and having a balanced lifestyle.

Ultimately, anyone makes lifestyle changes only by acting on new thoughts from a changed attitude and changed beliefs starting with an open mind.

Gratitude is so powerful with happy thinking. Good health could be said to be temporary, so being grateful today is important as it could all change tomorrow in an instant.

Getting to step 12 has nothing to do with age and

is best complemented by reviewing each step again.

Being reminded of the starting point through someone else who is suffering in denial, or beginning step one, and seeing them enjoy their improvements is very rewarding too. It is an ongoing wakeup call about having the privilege of choosing a healthy lifestyle and no longer being in denial of my addiction as a suffering chemaholic.

Here are ten points my fellow chemaholics and I arrived at when discussing how to spread a good message to anyone who is interested.

- Avoid arguments; they achieve nothing except waste valuable time. Only discussions with respectful listening achieve useful outcomes.

- Never be judgemental about a person's food nutrition beliefs. Ultimately, only the person can be deeply motivated to change his or her own beliefs through having reliable information and finding his or her own level of freedom.

- Be a good example – not a perfect one – offer inspiration at appropriate times.

- Offer a hand of help but do not grab victims as hostages.

- Give honest suggestions calmly and confidently when asked, pointing people in a direction for them to explore at their own pace.

• Offer understanding that a chemaholic lifestyle began as a voluntary choice without awareness then later turned into a physical and psychological need and, for those reasons, carries no blame.

• When someone asks for useful information but sound uninterested afterwards, continue offering it when asked again.

• Do not seek out compliments to artificially boost ego. However, when they come, humbly acknowledge the genuine ones with thanks and aim to learn something new in the process when possible.

• Compliment other people when they are making progress, however small the progress.

• Keep in contact with an open heart for fellow recovering chemaholics who may one day require to be supported as they may in turn support you.

First aid and saving lives

To have good first aid is important when it is urgently needed. It can be life saving. It is also very rewarding to know you have saved a life through a small amount of preparation. When someone you love needs urgent first aid the cost of preparation is really worth it.

Check first aid kits at home, car, work, holiday luggage always have several big bandages. Sometimes ambulances and hospitals are not always the fasted option when minutes count. This may be due to:

- Staffing levels

- Weather

- Financial constraints

- An unusual busy period

- The telephone operator taking too long or misunderstands

- Unexpected telephone or computer technical faults

If it is possible to be self sufficient with first aid it helps take off the financial pressure from the busy NHS.

How about take it to the next level and donate blood locally twice a year to help save lives. More information about registering for donations can be found at www.blood.co.uk. This also gives the donor a health test. Blood pressure and haemoglobin levels (iron) are checked at the time of the donation.

There are many first aid courses available free or low cost. One college I worked at paid for my course and appointed me as a first aider with a small pay increase.

There are easy to use gadgets available to check blood pressure, blood glucose and heart rate. These may be useful during first aid or simply for a quick personal at home health check for you and other people.

Summary

Step 12 maybe automatic for many people who have experienced a significantly healthier lifestyle over several months. There is a lot of joy in sharing something good with people who are ready to receive it.

I find it therapeutic to be reminded about my old beliefs. I aim to continue appreciating the value of being open minded on my journey. Increasing my awareness of each step helps my happy recovering chemaholic lifestyle.

Encouraging everyone to keep asking the right questions about food sources is so important to keep up personal learning. Many people ask the wrong questions so they get the wrong answers. For example:

- Is this healthy?

- Does it look healthy?

- Does it smell healthy?

- Does the texture and taste feel healthy enough to trust?

- Is the supplier well known?

There are many adverts for food and drinks which pre answer these questions in the advert with a "yes." The most valuable questions and answers come from asking about nutrition levels originating in the food source.

"Chemicalism was given to me as an inspiration. Making the word Chemicalism is my gift of truth. Sharing this truth is my service to other people."

Quiz Questions

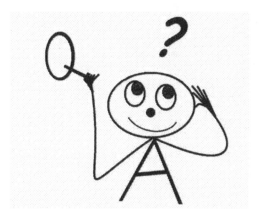

"Asking the right questions about nutrition sources provides quality answers."

To test your knowledge and keep you thinking about your health, have a go at these quick questions that are separated into age groups. The answers are easy to look up in the A – Z terms section.

The first essential step to a lifestyle change is having an open mind and developing a new habit of continuous questioning. This is a fun way to stimulate our ongoing awareness of chemicalism, uncovering a more in-depth awareness of natural nutrition.

The information we rely upon controls our decisions about our nutrition choices, which is all based on a lifetime of answered questions.

For example, I used to believe strongly that drinking a lot of water is healthy. When I explained this to my naturally healthy friend Elsa who has followed naturopathy for a life time, she said I was crazy! "Drinking water to excess without a thirst! "This meant my body was being over worked to process the over consumption of water. Initially, I defensively said that this good health message has been promoted everywhere and for years, quoting a few authoritative sources. Elsa looked at me with a puzzled expression and said after a slight pause," .... and you believe all that?"

However, I was extremely obese at the time, a suffering chemaholic. It was time to be open minded and question many preconceived notions. To be mentally ready for a change in lifestyle required a new questioning attitude every day and a check to see if my nutrition knowledge stood up to much deeper questioning.

Since 2013, I decided to drink water only when thirsty, listening to my body for natural signals, aiming for purified water when possible. Six months later in 2013, I became 22 kilos lighter from a combination of new lifestyle beliefs that have developed through quality questioning.

There are two routes our answers come from: either our own internal thoughts, sometimes intuition, or many types of external sources, especially commercial advertising and governmental promotion. Perhaps the best judge of the information to follow is the result shown and felt physically in the body.

The vast overload of changing external information we are given about healthy lifestyles would take too long to analyse with research, so it seems reasonable to believe without question what seems like the most rational. We trust authority that we believe is genuine. There are many examples of when it has taken several years for the truth to come to the surface publically about products with high toxicity .For example, all of these practices used to be acceptable: taking heroin for headaches, smoking cigarettes to relax, over consuming of alcohol to feel happy. Now, various, popular, medically prescribed drugs have been withdrawn, some artificial food dyes banned, along with asbestos in roofs, lead in water pipes, and air and water pollution from industrial waste. At one time, the majority of people believed all these things were good based on external information.

Every month, more external truth is coming to light about what the mass population consumes. I suggest that everyone keep questioning three levels deep about the true origins of what you consume, or to which you are exposed, building a more reliable internal source of reference.

It takes only a few moments to check the EXTERNAL INFORMATION on the packaging for the ingredients. Then, you should reflect with your INTERNAL INFORMATION, using good quality questions such as: did the product get sprayed with pesticides? is there a very long list of artificial chemicals included that may not be required? what does " free from " mean?

Children and Kids

1 Where do chips come from?

2 What is the vitamin we receive naturally from being in the sun light?

3 Which main vitamin does an orange give you?

4 What percentage of our body is water?

5 Why does mains tap water require weed killer to be added so it is able to reach the taps inside homes from the main pumping station?

6 What is the natural life expectancy of a cow?

7 What is an "E" number or food number tell you on the packaging of   manufactured food & drink products sold in shops?

8 What is processed food?

9 What is organic food and drink?

10 Where does lactose come from?

11 Where does gluten come from?

12 Where does real natural salt come from?

Teenagers

1 Does natural fruit contain sugar?

2 How long after consuming sugary sweets or drinks do you expect to feel more energy from a sugar high?

3 Why does a sugar high give you an appetite to consume more sugary foods and drinks soon after?

4 Does smoking cause cancer?

5 Why do people need to be vaccinated?

6 What words do the illness abbreviations H.I.V.or AIDS stand for?

7 Is a food or drink allergy the same as intolerance?

8 Where does real live probiotic yoghurt come from?

9 What poison do alcoholic drinks contain which are also used as an industrial cleaner?

10 What does a person die of if they drink only salty sea water?

11 Do foods with a high amount of salt make a person become more thirsty?

12 Why is mass produced sugar normally white?

Adults

1 Do all fish sold in super markets grow up naturally in the sea, river and lakes?

2 As vegetables lose their nutrition when stored in the open, does freezing vegetables lock in their nutrition?

3 What is the cooking method that gives maximum nutrition from organic vegetables: boiled, deep fried, pressure cooked, microwave or grilled?

4 How long after eating does it take for the chemicals in our stomach to tell the brain how full it is as the food is being digested?

5 Is reflux (a feeling of food coming back up from the stomach) mainly caused shortly after rapidly gulping down highly processed (non organic) foods and drinks?

6 Are lemons acid or alkaline when inside us after we have eaten them?

7 What is the chemical additive E621 Monosodium Glutamate abbreviated "MSG" used for in food?

8 Why do people become over weight due to lack of sleep?

9 Why does the brain shrink by 60% at night?

10 Which organic milk has higher nutrition: skimmed or full fat?

11 How does the food digestive process first get started when we eat?

12 What is the source/s of low priced bottled water sold in shops that do not state the source as spring or mineral?

Seniors

1 What vitamin would you lack when staying permanently indoors away from the sunlight?

2 Is it good practice to wash food with tap water?

3 After taking a course of doctor prescribed tablet antibiotics which kill both bad and good bacteria, is it helpful to consume some kind of probiotic to regenerate natural good bacteria quickly?

4 What (UK) legal approval mark on food packaging means you avoid consuming pesticides sprayed on low cost vegetables and fruit?

5 Blood pressure normally increases with age. Are natural herbs such as garlic and ginger able to reduce blood pressure?

6 Is it possible to recover from Diabetes Type II after 90 years of age by swapping to a high nutrition natural food and drink lifestyle?

7 Is it possible to recover from terminal gangrene after 90 years of age by swapping to a high nutrition natural food and drink lifestyle?

8 Is it possible to recover / reduce from high bad cholesterol numbers after 90 years of age by swapping to a high nutrition, natural food and drink lifestyle?

9 What medically approved, scientifically proven electrical gadgets are available for personal use to improve circulation and remove or reduce pain to help maintain good joint movements?

10 Are chemical isotonic vitamin supplements more likely to be absorbed into the body?

11 Where is the best place to find published information about appetite side effects for prescribed medication?

12 Why is Manuka Honey so good at healing the body naturally?

Terms & Quiz Question Answers

Acupuncture is an external treatment using very fine needles to stimulate meridian energy points in the body. The success of this treatment to cure many health conditions has lasted over several hundred years. It has been proven to cure all kinds of un-wellness both physical and emotional. Most towns in The UK have a private treatment centre.

AIDS is a virus acquired by infection that results in a low immunity allowing a wide range of different diseases and opportunistic infections.

Acquired Immune Deficiency Syndrome.

Alcohol is a strong toxic liquid used as an industrial and medical cleaner which also kill germs. Describing a person who has over consumed alcoholic drinks is called "intoxicated" Only a small percentage of alcohol is legally permitted to be added in drinks that are retailed. Drinking pure alcohol can cause blindness. The liver is good at processing the alcohol toxins but over time the function of the liver is decreased. Moderation is the key to allow enjoyment. Drinking alcohol after food normally reduces the side effects.

Allergies are stronger than intolerances. Allergies can be life threatening in some cases which require immediate medication.

Building up natural immunity with a high nutrition lifestyle may help reduce the risks of some allergies.

Ambushing is a surprise attack strategy to gain advantage by tricking the opponent. In relation to this book it means using multiple methods to produce improved health.

Amino Acids are very important, our body does not produce all of them so we obtain them from natural food. Suffering chemaholics may require a general amino acid supplement to help kick start their recovery process at the beginning of a lifestyle change as well as ongoing well-ness.

Addiction is a mental and or physical state. An addict needs to frequently repeat a habit or type of behaviour even when the known outcome causes an unpleasant withdrawal. The start of a long term addiction recovery is a change in attitude.

Adrenaline (Epinephrine) is produced by the human body when there is an immediate threat of death. The body reacts to adrenaline within minutes with air passages dilating, blood is redirected to the heart and lungs. This can be self injected using a pen. It is the first line of treatment for severe life-threatening allergic reactions. The best first aid kits contain two of the auto injector pens.

Amputation of limbs related to people suffering with diabetes II is on the increase as diabetes type II is on the increase. Diabetes type II is common for people suffering from obesity and poor nutrition. Circulation of blood around the body transporting the healing oxygen is essential to cure gangrene. Exercise however modest helps the circulation. My mum who had been diabetic type II recovered from diabetes during 2014 and no longer required an amputation. Circulation was helped in many ways including acupuncture.

Antibiotics prescribed by a medical professional are designed to kill bacteria which also mean both good and bad bacteria. After a course of prescribed antibiotics it is important to rebuild the good "friendly" bacteria using probiotics. Before modern day anti biotics there have been many natural antibiotics. For example Honey is considered a well known antibiotic.

Autointoxication is when the built up of undigested, stagnant waste in the colon starts to re-enter the body through the blood supply as a toxin causing all kinds of un-wellness.

Aversion therapy is a type of psychological treatment to overcome unwanted behaviour. By repeating the same behaviour over again with a negative outcome the behaviour becomes uninteresting. This therapy can be used with some addictions. For example smoking one hundred cigarettes every day for one week may take away an addiction to smoking when the behaviour is associated with feeling sick.

Appetite describes a mental state of a noticeable desire or craving to receive something typically food. With Chemicalism it applies to a suffering chemaholic craving a mood uplift by wanting to consume chemaholic food and drinks. Increased food and drink appetite can be stimulated by artificial chemicals such as MSG; natural chemicals salt; and many prescribed drugs. A natural appetite can be stimulated by exercise. It is better to eat and drink in response to natural feelings of hunger and thirst.

Aromatherapy is a therapeutic method using smells. These are usually commercially in the form of essential oils and can be used for all kinds of un-wellness. For example anti-depressant, sleeping, memory, relaxation.

Bees pollinate around a third of what humans eat. They are essential to the worlds ecosystem. They eat only nectar and pollen from flowers and plants. The plants require bees to reproduce. Bees produce honey of different qualities. Manuka honey is among the best in the world and has many healing properties for internal and external uses.

Bloated in terms of a suffering chemaholic describes the swelling in the digestive system. This is due to eating faster than the digestive system has had time to report back to the brain that it has a feeling of fullness. For some people it is the inflammation caused in the persons digestive system by the chemaholic food. As everyone has different levels of intolerance to artificial chemicals the level of bloating varies a lot.

Blood pressure needs to be at the right level to make the body work properly. There are natural remedies to reduce blood pressure which include many advertised herbs such ginger and garlic. Like all foods some people can have intolerances and allergies to even the advertised nature cures. It is best to get intolerance and allergy tests to confirm the best natural remedies. There are many prescribed medicines to control blood pressure; it is a good idea to check the manufacturer's published side effects.

It is possible to test blood pressure at home with a small gadget that gives an instant result. This is a useful addition to a first aid kit.

Blood tests are normally carried out by a nurse. One sample can be used to carry out many tests. A doctor usually ticks the boxes on a form to choose only certain tests are required. These tests can typically be:

- blood cholesterol test
- blood culture
- blood gases test
- blood glucose (blood sugar) tests
- blood typing
- cancer blood tests
- chromosome testing (karyotyping)
- coagulation tests and international normalised ratio (INR)
- C-reactive protein (CRP) test
- electrolyte test
- erythrocyte sedimentation rate (ESR)
- full blood count (FBC)
- genetic testing and screening
- liver function test
- thyroid function test

The glucose test is possible to carry out at home with a small gadget that gives an instant result. This is helpful for diabetics or borderline diabetics to monitor glucose levels and assist with first aid diagnosis.

BMI stands for an international medical standard Body Mass Index. By taking height, weight, gender and age a BMI number is calculated. The BMI number indicates how healthy a person is:

18.5 – 24.9   Ideal weight

25 – 29.9   Overweight

30 – 39.9   Obese

40+   Very obese

There are some other personal factors which may alter an average reading such as muscular people will have a heavier weight.

Brain detoxing occurs when the body is asleep as the brain reduces in size by around 60% allowing brain specific chemicals to engage a cleaning process. Step 11 explains more.

Calorie is a unit of measurement of energy that comes from consuming nutrition in food and drinks. This energy is used up with exercise and essential basic functions of the body. The amount of calories used in a human body to carry out the basic functions is called your basal metabolic rate (metabolism) and accounts for around 70% of calorie burning:

The basic functions of the body (basal metabolic rate) includes:

- Breathing
- Blood circulating
- Adjusting levels of hormones
- Growing and repairing cells

Knowing 70% of calories are automatically burnt off naturally which rarely alters, means only the remaining 30% is down to food types and exercise. I believe by consuming 80% of natural foods the body does not struggle with burning off some artificial chemicals. I believe this explains why recovering chemaholics have an increased physical energy to burn off calories from natural foods.

Marketing of low nutrition products often advertises low calorie content and not the metabolic burn off rate which may be misleading in many cases.

Cancer cells are generated in the body everyday and with high immunity the body manages these new cancer cells to stop them multiplying. The right level of natural nutrition is essential to be absorbed into the body. Reliable advise is promoted by The World Health Organisation (WHO) and Cancer Research UK www.cancerhelp. org.uk   There are cancer help charities in most countries offering lots of free advice about the different causes.

Carbohydrates see nutrition

Chemaholic describes a person or animal suffering from Chemicalism. A Chemaholic has:

- Regular compulsive cravings or binge cravings
- Loss of control over the consumption
- Despite negative consequences and withdrawal upon stopping consumption
- Both rewarding and reinforcing
- May not be aware they are a Chemaholic of processed food and drinks made or grown with Artificial Chemicals.

Chemicalism The subject of artificial Chemically processed food and drink addictive dependence by Human beings and animals.

Chewing food is about the first stage of digestion as the chemicals in the mouth are activated usually by smell and thoughts. The physical breaking down of food with the enzymes from the mouth is essential for easily absorbing the nutrition as it passes to the second stage.

Chips are sliced potatoes fried in oil Potatoes grow in the ground. One tasty natural alternative is organic potatoes avoiding pesticides, not washed in tap water containing chemicals, sliced thickly, fried in a natural cooking oil.

Chiropractor is a professionally qualified person who treats people with muscular disorders in the spine or joints which require manual manipulation. A good chiropractor will reduce or cure pain then improve functionality of the joints when possible. After the main adjustment is put right it is often followed up with physiotherapy.

Cholesterol is often mentioned in a bad way as being too high and shown up in blood tests. Both myself and my mum's (94 years) reduced cholesterol levels to normal levels within six months of changing to an 80% natural nutrition lifestyle. There is a lot of research that can be read up on cholesterol to become expert. Instead perhaps it is easier to focus on just enjoying the benefits of natural foods first and decide if you have time to study cholesterol in more detail later.

Circulation Booster machine using TENS technology. Electrical gadgets using tiny electrical impulses stimulate the circulation. The body complains with aches and pains signalling where the problem area is in need of help. My mum started using one of these gadgets at 93 years. The electrical stimulation brought back the use in my mum's fingers. This meant she could enjoy chopping up vegetables having not been able to do so for many years. I have used the same machine to help re grow a served nerve in my leg

_ motorcycle accident.

Cognitive dissonance is a psychological term to describe the personal stress of having two conflicting beliefs, or values at the same time. In the 12 steps there are likely to be many times when this is experienced when giving up lifetime habits justified by old unhelpful values which are the opposite of strong beliefs.

Contaminants in water vary from country to country and locally to the supply of mains unfiltered tap water. Government regulations provide water supply companies with minimum standards. There is no guarantee the raw tap water is without contaminants unless you have a 99%+ filter method in place. The water board standards are very high in most European countries but it is not perfect. Many water companies claim they offer 99% of clean water in line with government standards but this is not 99% filtered.

Be aware supermarket bottled water not containing mineral or spring water is tap water. The plastic bottled water industry thriving due to the general awareness unfiltered tap water can be improved.

Colloidal Silver is a natural anti-biotical remedy. My mum used it to spray on her feet to reduce inflammation. It is purified water and silver. The Greek and Romans empires used it to provide immunity. NASA used a silver system on the Space Shuttle. Also my mum drank purified water at home from a pure silver cup to assist with overcoming terminal gangrene.

Colon therapy (Colonic) is a detoxification method of the large intestine by two methods:

- Oral products from chemists, health shops and online which can contain natural ingredients. These tablets and solutions are often taken over a few days. Some people simply use an enema or laxative.

- A cleaning process using water under gentle pressure pumped and released into the rectum by a qualified professional. Some therapists add probiotics to generate new good bacteria and herbs to enhanced the clearing process. A treatment usually takes one hour.

After clearing the built up waste encrusted on the colon walls it is claimed to improve immunity, increase physical energy and produce a feeling of mental well-being. I agree with these claims although there are few studies to confirm this.

Dr. John Harvey Kellogg at the Battle Creek Sanatorium, who 'maintained that 90% of the diseases of civilization are due to improper functioning of the colon.'

Once the colon has been cleaned out ongoing management with plant based nutrition and probiotics to strengthen the good bacteria help immunity.

Constipation This is commonly caused by diets with low fibre and high levels of chemaholic foods that are difficult to digest. Common chemaholic symptoms include headaches, bloating, tiredness, bad breath and producing foul smelling wind. This unwell-ness is rarely found in people consuming mainly plant based diets. With constipation being more of a lifestyle habit most people understand this condition as IBS irritable bowl syndrome. (see **autointoxication**.)

Cooking organic vegetables and other natural foods in a steam cooker locks in the maximum amount of nutrition avoiding it to boil off.

Cows naturally live up to 20 -25 years. Cows living through an intensive commercial farming process are feed with artificial chemical foods. This encourages quicker growth; high milk production but the cows's life span is reduced to typically 4 – 5 years.

Counselling or talking therapies have many different specialist types to overcome troubling emotions for example bereavement, relationships, addictions. The common type practised in the UK involves a patient talking about their past to a therapist. Most top professionals including athletes tend to have motivational counselling or coaching which focuses on how to achieve goals. This long term solution therapy is not always available to patients and often medications are the prescribed alternative.

Deprivation in terms of this 12 step chemaholic recovery plan means enjoying around 80% of natural, mainly organic nutrition and 20% of any other nutrition to avoid feelings of guilt or deprivation.

Detoxing (detoxification) or Detox as a shortened slang. This is a widely used term and generally means filtering out the poisons which are toxic from the body. This is normally a natural process happening 24 hours a day using the body organs when they are working correctly.

Over consumption of alcohol causes intoxication. There are many poisons that are toxic such as certain chemaholic foods and drinks, heroine, lead and rust from water pipes. Natural growing fungi that is similar to mushrooms. Pollution within the air from engine fumes. The list is long so with so many modern day poisons the body organs are under extra pressure to perform.

There are many short term detoxing solutions to help clean up the organs. The best detoxing approach is a happy lifestyle change providing a strong natural daily filtering maintenance.

Diabetes Type I (one) used to be called insulin dependent diabetes. It is when there is a lack of insulin produced by the body. Doctors provide patients with insulin to be injected usually multiple times each day.

Diabetes Type II is the most common type and many people manage it with healthy food nutrition. My mum recovered from Diabetes Type II at 94 years old after changing to a natural high nutrition lifestyle. This could be said overcomes the theory of becoming diabetic just due to older age. Doctors offer tablets to control type II diabetes. My mum recovered from Diabetes type II having reduced medications from the un-wellness. Therefore it could be said I am no longer at risk genetically suggesting nutrition lifestyle may overcome the inherited genetic theory.

Diarrhoea is one of the natural ways the body reacts when attempting to clear something that it has detected as harmful. Too much diarrhoea lasting over 24 hours can turn into dehydration due to fluid loss. There is a long list of causes many to do with digestion, inflammation, food allergies & intolerances, over consumption toxins e.g. of alcohol, food poisoning.

Digestion starts with smell triggering digestive juices. The mouth uses a combination of mechanical chewing and chemicals to break down the food before the next process. I feel it is worth adding that thinking about favourite foods when hungry can also trigger the digestive chemicals in the mouth from my experience.

It takes 15 – 20 minutes for the digestive chemicals to tell the brain how full the stomach has become.

The main process of digestion is:

Sight & smell   Salivation

Mouth   Chewing and saliva digestive juices break down starches

Oesophagus   Swallowing

Stomach   Upper relaxes to let food enter

                 Lower mixes food with digestive juice

                 Stomach acid breaks down Protein

Small intestine Peristalsis movement

                 Digestive juice breaks down starches, protein, carbohydrates

Pancreas	Pancreatic juice Starches breaks down fats protein
Liver	Bile acids digestive juices breaks down Fats

Digestive enzymes get to work on the food we eat and turn it into nutrients so the body is able to absorb the nutrition. Eating the highest nutrition food is of little value when there is not enough digestive enzymes in the body to absorb the nutrition.

Chronic stress is the most common reason for lack of digestive enzymes and therefore inability to absorb nutrition. The body has two states:

- Sympathetic "fight or flight" digestion is given very low priority so digestive enzyme output is very low

- Parasympathetic "rest and digest" allows high absorption of nutrition because the maximum digestive enzymes are used to break down the food.

Symptoms suggesting the digestive enzymes are not working fully include the chemaholic bloating after meals and foul smelling gas.

There are isotonic supplements to provide digestive enzymes some include probiotics for adults and children. A high quality isotonic supplement is a way to kick start increased nutrition especially in step one.

Dopamine functions as a neurotransmitter, a chemical released by neurons to send signals to other nerve cells the brain. Dopamine plays a role in the way our brain controls movements. Parkinson's disease patients have low dopamine with the person losing their ability to execute smooth, controlled movements.

Both serotonin and dopamine increase your mood of happiness.

It is possible to increase dopamine through:

Natural nutrition

- Dopamine boosting supplements
- Physical exercise
- Meditation
- harmful drug addictions such as cocaine

Dopamine makes us feel good. It helps control weight, energy levels, supports brain functions such as memory and contributes to a healthy heart. Otherwise without out it, we would be fat, unhappy, and tired.

Since dopamine is synthesized from an amino acid tyrosine, you can eat foods rich in tyrosine to boost dopamine production. Phenylalnine is an essential amino acid which converts in the body to tyrosine. Certain foods help balance dopamine levels, including:

- Apples
- Fish
- Eggs
- Bananas
- Spirulina
- Red beets
- Kale
- Oregano Oil
- Herbs ginkgo biloba,

  ginseng
- Turmeric
- Avocados
- Chocolate
- Strawberries and blueberries
- Green tea
- Coffee
- Nuts Seeds

"E" numbers are food ingredient chemical references numbers beginning with "E" then a number. They define an additive to foods made in Europe (since 1962) such as food colourings and MSG. In non European countries such as USA they follow a similar system without the "E". Standards differ outside Europe, some chemicals are banned in Europe but allowed in other countries. There is a list at www.chemicalism.org

Electrolytes are all about keeping the body running with electrical voltage levels being constant through our kidneys and several hormones. Exercising produces sweat so we lose electrolytes, mainly potassium and sodium.

We keep the electrolyte concentrations in our body fluids, by eating fruits and vegetables which have a good sources of sodium and potassium to replace lost electrolytes. Too much electrolyte levels in the blood stream get filtered out by the kidneys.

Flatulence is passing gas, from the digestive system out of the anus. One cause is eating quickly and taking in extra air. Carbonated drinks may cause a build up of gas. Some foods the human body is not designed to absorb so they pass from the intestines to the colon without proper digestion. In the colon the bacteria breaks down the food with bacteria which releases gases.

Freezing foods locks in there nutrition and stops the natural process of decay. Vegetables lose their nutrition when stored in the open air.

Fish can grow up naturally in the sea and rivers. Also they can be grown in fish farms and feed on chemically enhanced food to increase their size quickly. Both sea and river water can have a percentage of toxins in it. The smaller fish with shorter life spans have less time to absorb toxins.

Food digestion starts with the digestive chemicals produced in the mouth which of often the result of smelling the food. The chewing of food is very important to get the digestive chemicals to begin working on breaking down the food ready for the next stage.

Gangrene occurs through lack of blood circulating around the body carrying oxygen. When the ends of toes, fingers, feet, hands lack circulation the infection starts. The normal medical remedy to avoid death is to amputate the gangrene area to stop it spreading plus antibiotics. However in the case of my mum in 2014 she had recovered from terminal gangrene after changing to a natural nutrition lifestyle.

Gout is a form of arthritis, affecting joints with swelling and pain in my case it was both feet. I no longer have gout it has completely cured after a month of not drinking red wine and eating mainly homemade vegetable soup.

Glucose is a sugar providing an essential energy source for all the cells and organs of our body including our muscles and brain. Glucose comes from the food we eat. Carbohydrates in fruit, bread pasta and cereals are common sources of glucose. Small gadgets can be used at home to test glucose levels.

Gluten is found in wheat, barley and rye grains. Some people have an intolerance or allergy towards gluten and may choose gluten free food and drinks. The cows that produce the milk are not pastured, they are gluten fed. It is possible to buy gluten free milk and cheese.

Gut functions include digestion. It is widely understood to have an ability that gives human beings a basic instinct of intuition. "a gut reaction"

Many people treat their guts as a bit of mysterious plumbing rather than respect its fine tuned intelligence.

This complex organ like the brain is complex whilst it processes foods with bacteria, measuring salt, absorbing nutrients.

Over 90% of the body's serotonin lives in the gut, the remainder in the brain. Serotonin is a chemical that is involved with happiness levels, sex, sleeping. This suggests the gut has a big influence over how happy a person feels.

It has up to 100 million neurons, a similar amount found in the spinal cord plus about 40 neurotransmitters similar to the amount in the brain. The Gut has a high level of intelligence.

Amazingly when the main vagus nerve connecting the gut to the brain is cut, the gut is cleverly able to continue working independently of the brain and spinal cord!

HEPA filters "High Efficiency Particulate Arrestance" are used to filter or detox the air and are found in aircrafts and hospitals. They were invented in 1940 to take out airborne radioactive contaminants. Nowadays they are available in retail stores and online. HEPA filters are specially made to target very small pollutants and particles.

H.I.V. Human Immuneodeficiency Virus attacks the white blood cells which naturally fight off disease. A person testing HIV positive does not mean they have AIDS; it can take around 10–12 years to progress to AIDS.

Once HIV is diagnosed before it becomes AIDS, there are medicines which slowdown or stop the damage to the immune system. If AIDS then develops, medicines can usually help the immune system become healthier.

There are two types of HIV:

- HIV-1 being almost all the cases of AIDS worldwide
- HIV-2 is an AIDS-like illness. Uncommon in North America.

Without a strong immune system, the body has trouble fighting off disease which can lead to all kinds of un-wellness including cancer.

Homeopathy is a natural medicine to treat both acute and chronic un-wellness. It is based on the principle of 'like cures like'. This means, a substance taken in small amounts will cure the same symptoms it causes if it were taken in large amounts by building up a tolerance.

It uses a whole body, holistic approach with each person treated as a unique individual body, mind, spirit and emotions are all considered. Prevention of disease and self healing is the aim. These medicines rarely cause any side-effects and best results come from consulting with a qualified homeopath.

Himalayan bath salts used in bathing in a bath allows the skin to absorb the salts natural trace minerals whilst detoxing the skin at the same time. There are many medicinal benefits of natural Himalayan bath salts which have been a medicine for several thousand years. They are said to be the most purist of sea salt and coming from the Himalayan Mountains. (The skin is the largest organ of the body.)

Hydrotherapy (water therapy) was one of the very first natural therapies. This is using the flow of water in different ways. This includes putting your feet in a running stream. However the modern day alternative is often to visit a leisure centre and sit in a Jacuzzi. There are many water bubbling hydrotherapy options for use at home to promote a feeling of well being and improve circulation.

Intolerance to certain foods, drinks, smells and skin absorbed substances cause an uncomfortable reaction such as a rash, nausea, lack of energy, headaches, the list is very long. These are not life threatening. I have seen many people become free or reduce their intolerances a few weeks after just swapping to purified water. Building up your natural immunity with a high nutrition lifestyle may help take away intolerances or reduce the reaction. Having a food test is wise because quickly you are able to understand what your body is designed to process. Review this after several weeks of changing to a natural food lifestyle can find out if the intolerances have gone. (See Allergies)

IBS irritable bowl syndrome is caused by the digestive system being fed the wrong food. Suffering chemaholics have periods of:

- Diarrhoea (with foul smells)
- Constipation and flatulence
- Stomach bloating cramping pain
- Feeling of sickness
- Backache
- Bad smelling breath

There are many fast acting non prescription tablets to stop the symptoms. Hospital tests, blood tests usually show there is no medical condition to treat such as cancer but it is good to rule it out. Good doctors offer nutrition advice. Exercise is not a cure.

Immunity is low for suffering chemaholics who often have many food intolerances due to low immunity; catching colds and infections is regularly is normal. Strong immunity is maintained with a high nutrition food and drink lifestyle avoiding intolerant or allergic products.

Isotonic vitamin supplements are claimed to be better because they are absorbed into the body faster in a liquid form with a higher percentage of the nutrition being absorbed. They are usually more expensive and come in a power form.

Lactose sugar is in cow's milk. Some people have an intolerance or allergy towards Lactose. There are many alternative natural options made with soya, rice and nuts. Checking the ingredients of the alternatives is always a good idea; some have been processed, some have sugars or artificial sweeteners added.

Koala (nicknamed Koala Bear) is a mammal sleeping 18 to 22 a day due to a low nutrition high toxic, high fibre diet of Australian eucalyptus leaves. They rarely drink and the origin of their name is from the Aboriginal language meaning "do not need to drink"   www.savethekoala.com

Libido or sex drive level is normally referred to as being high or low. It is driven by psychological and biological instincts. There are many factors such as stress, exercise levels, drug side effects, un-wellness through being a suffering chemaholic that may reduce libido. A high nutrition life style allows the body a good chance of functioning well psychologically and biologically.

Lifestyle change means a for life way of living. This seems to have taken over from the negative phase of slimming diets which normally fails after a few weeks or months because they are usually too inconvenient therefore unsustainable. The ultimate lifestyle is a psychologically happy one with high nutrition foods and some exercise being at the core. When changing from a low nutrition chemaholic lifestyle to high nutrition it is best to do this gradually over several weeks so the body adjusts smoothly.

Lemons well known for providing vitamin C they are acid but when consumed by humans turn to alkaline which is healthy for the body.

Lymph Nodes are glands throughout the body providing immunity. They make up the gland system which carries nutrients and waste material between body tissues and bloodstream. The lymph nodes filter fluids trapping viruses, bacteria and foreign substances which are destroyed by white blood cells.

Manuka Honey has always been known as originating from New Zealand. Honey is made by bees. Manuka honey has many antibacterial healing properties.

Malabsorption syndrome covers a number of medical disorders when the intestine does not fully absorb nutrients into the bloodstream. This means nutrition is not absorbed from macronutrients ; proteins, carbohydrates; fats or micronutrients vitamins and minerals. See Digestive Enzymes.

Massage of the body has many benefits from detoxing points, relaxing, improving circulation and helping a general feeling of well-being.

- Reflexology
- Indian head massage
- Swedish Massage Therapy
- Hot Stone Massage
- Deep Tissue Massage
- Thai massage manipulation
- Pregnancy massage
- Aromatherapy

Many people spend several hours a day sitting continuously at a computer or screen which tightens the neck and back muscles. There are many gadgets to provide a neck massage to release the stress at the top of the spine.

The body needs to be relaxed for the best digestion to take place and massage is another important method of ambushing the body with wellness.

Milk is produced by animals for their baby to feed on. Industrial production of milk on a large scale is made by cows by inducing a state of pregnancy using industrial foods to boost milk production. Humans also drink goats' milk. There are many alternatives to cow's milk designed for a baby cow (calves.) Alternative drinks made from Soya Beans, various nuts and rice. A lot of dairy milk has been pasteurised so the goodness is extracted. Full fat organic milk has the richest nutrition. Many people cannot consume cows milk due to being lactose intolerant.

Mindfulness is about paying deliberate attention in a specific way, on purpose, in the present moment. In terms of this book it means being aware at the moment of eating food and the immediate feedback from the physical body. For example being sure what the ingredients are in the meal, chewing the food many times perhaps 100 then sensing when the body is feeling full. When relaxing peacefully, even meditating considering how the body is giving out physical messages to be listened to for example a headache in a specific place.

Minerals are inorganic elements that come from the soil and water and are absorbed by plants or eaten by animals. By having a food intolerance test it will show up the best foods to works with your body.

Monosodium Glutamate E621 is an artificial chemical used for food flavouring enhancement. Some manufacturer labels do not list an E number instead it states "flavour enhancer" Other names, There are other E numbers which are associated with the MSG chemical.

MRI Scans Magnetic resonance imaging is the best and most expensive way to get clear detailed images of soft tissue inside the body. Glands can be looked at from all directions and in colour. MRI scans are not so good at imaging bones because of the lower water content. As MRI scanning is not available for everyone alternative diagnosis tests include:

- Computed tomography (CT)
- X-ray scan
- Ultrasound
- Blood test
- Biopsy

It is important to get the best health checks available, some of them are free.

Nauru is a small island in The pacific ocean recording in 2012 the population has an obesity rate of 71.7 % also this little republic country recorded the highest population with type 2 diabetes making up around 40 % of the population.

Natural Food for the purpose of this book means organic without artificial chemicals:

- Vegetables
- Fruit
- Meat
- Fish
- Products or living creatures /beings grown or harvested without artificial chemicals
- Foods and drinks made from natural sources without a major reduction in nutrition due to a process

Naturopathy is a combination of natural self healing methods unique to each person. It looks to discover the cause of a condition and not suppress it. A holistic; whole body approach means not just looking at one organ that is being affected. There are several governing bodies regulating the qualifications for naturopathic professionals listed at www.gncouncil.co.uk

Nutrition is the process of absorbing nutrients from foods eaten. The foods we choose determines which nutrients will be used to:

- Make energy
- Regulate the processes of the body
- Build and maintain tissues

The first three of the six types of nutrients are called macronutrients because they are required in large quantities

- Carbohydrates
- Lipids
- Proteins
- Water
- Vitamins
- Minerals

The macronutrients carbohydrates, lipids and proteins are the only nutrients providing your body with energy, which is measured in calories.

Carbohydrates provide quick energy because they are readily available when there is an immediate need for energy. Carbohydrates come from food. There are different foods containing different types of carbohydrates. For example, a biscuit is mainly sugars, this is a simple carbohydrate. Spaghetti contains a lot of starches, which are complex carbohydrates composed of many sugars. Fruits and vegetables provide fiber, which is a type of carbohydrate that cannot be digested. This means you do not get energy from fiber. Fiber is needed for moving foods through the digestive system.

Lipids or fats, have more calories per gram than all other macronutrients. They are energy dense nutrients providing sustainable energy when you require some endurance. There are different types of fats. Saturated fats, like butter, are solid at room temperature; unsaturated fats, like vegetable oils, are liquid at room temperature. Fats are good to aid weight loss which include avocados, nuts and fish.

Proteins contain calories and proteins are so important for growth, development and repair, the body uses them as a last resort source of energy. Proteins come from animal and plant foods. The body breaks these protein containing foods down into amino acids. The amino acids then get reassembled into many different types of body proteins.

Water is a nutrient. Unlike the other nutrients, it is a single substance. It is easily lost through sweat, urine, sweat and evaporation. This means regular drinks when thirsty; eating foods containing water, fruits and vegetables. Water lubricates joints, transports substances around the body regulating body temperature.

Micronutrients are the opposite of macronutrients which come in small quantities. Vitamins and minerals, are micronutrients which do not contain calories, as they do not directly provide your body with energy.

The main functions of vitamins are

- Energy metabolism, converting calorie-containing nutrients into energy
- Maintaining vision
- Protecting cells from damage
- Helping with blood clotting

Vitamins can be either fat soluble(stored in fatty tissues) or water soluble so they dissolve in water then are easily flushed out of the body.

Obesity Obese describes the level of having excess weight in relation to body height. A BMI (Body Mass Index) over 30 indicates a person who is obese and suffering from obesity. The BMI scale is an internationally accepted method of measuring obesity.

Oranges contain vitamin "C" it is better to consume organic oranges to avoid consuming pesticides which are sprayed onto the oranges to maximise the harvest.

Organic Foods are natural food & drink without pesticides sprayed on fruit, vegetables, no artificial growth chemicals feed to the livestock. No artificial chemicals added.

ORGANIC LABELLED foods are made from natural sources without artificial chemicals which have been approved by a government standard agency issuing licences to use the organic label. These government standards differ in different countries. There is a difference between the UK and USA.

Organ systems are complex with 12 of them. The four main ones mentioned in this book are:

- Digestive
- Immune
- Reproductive
- Nervous

Organs in the human body are described briefly in step 8 with the main message that they all contain a high amount of water which is essential to the detoxing filtering process.(Blood contains 83% - bones 31%.)

These are the percentages of water in each organ

according to H.H. Mitchell, (1945) Journal of Biological Chemistry 158:

- Brain and spinal cord   73%
- Heart   73%
- Liver   71%
- Kidneys   79%
- Pancreas   73%
- Spleen   78%
- Lungs   83%
- Muscles   79%
- Skin   64%

Orthopaedic Consultants specialise in surgery of injuries and conditions related to:

- Bones
- Joints
- Ligaments
- Tendons
- Muscles
- Nerves

Osteopathy is a treatment provided by a trained professional to cure or reduce medical disorders through the manipulation and massage of the bones, joints, and muscles.

Pesticides kill insects on plants, crops often have many types sprayed on them to help bring a profitable harvest. Organic foods are not allowed to be sprayed with pesticides and are able to advertise this on their packaging as "Organic".

Probiotics are live bacteria, yeasts which are essential for good health, especially in the digestive system. Probiotics can be bought over the counter as a supplement, live ones are kept refrigerated. They can be made at home.

Placebo drugs and testing are used to test new drugs. A study group of patients suffering from a disease or other medical condition is split up with half the group taking the real drugs or treatment. The other half of the group takes a medically ineffectual treatment or drug. Some patients taking the placebo drugs or treatment show health improvements this is called the placebo effect.

Amazing research is now showing people who are told they are being given a drug that is a placebo before taking a course of placebo drugs are reporting they have become well !

Plant remedies and supplements there are many good products available that have stood the test of time which continuing selling in a thriving industry of natural remedies. However, to receive the commercial acknowledgement it requires big budgets to fund clinical trials. Therefore, many plant based non medical products for example reseveratrol and pycnogenol cannot make any health claims due to medical legislation. The good news is that these natural plant based remedies are available without prescription.

Processed Foods are any food that has been altered from its original natural state often this term is used in slang referring to food with added artificial chemicals. The best processed foods are made from organic and natural ingredients.

Q10 - Co-Q10 co-enzyme is similar to a vitamin. It is naturally produced for all the cells in the human body with the production of it decreasing with age. The body needs Q10 to growth and maintenance cells. Organs with the highest energy requirements are the heart, liver, and kidney which have the highest CoQ10 concentration

It functions as an antioxidant protecting the body from damage caused by harmful molecules. There is no published clinical research that CoQ10 cures cancer. It can be found in some foods such as sardines and mackerel. It can be purchased as supplement without prescription.

Oesophagitis inflammation is mostly caused by reflux of acid from the stomach. The food we eat goes down the gullet (oesophagus) into our stomach. A one way valve opens temporarily to let the food in. The cells in the stomach lining make chemicals and acid to digest the food as well as a mucus to protect the stomach from the acid.

When food refluxes back up the oesophagus the unpleasant stomach acid can be tasted on the back of the throat. The oesophagus's wall linings have little protection and become inflamed.

There are many over the counter non prescription medicines to reduce the inflammation which are commonly called heart burn medications.

Two ways this un-wellness occurs is eating large meals fast and laying down eating.

Reflexology is a natural treatment involving gentle massaging normally of the feet and hands to help increased wellness elsewhere in the body. This is considered by many people as detoxing. This therapy has not been given any scientific proof that it works but remains very popular as a therapy.

Reflux I think of as food having a difficult time being digested so the food starts to make its way back up the throat but not causing vomiting. Strong Reflux which is noticeable can be caused by lots reasons only one of them is gulping down food fast. Too much reflux can lead to a cough which sometimes can be mistaken as a chest infection. Common noticeable reflux symptoms are heart burn. Also see oesophagitis caused by inflammation.

Salt naturally comes from the evaporation of sea water for Sea salt and salt Mines under the ground. Natural salt is usually more expensive to buy than laboratory produced cheap table salt.

The low cost table salt has been stripped of the natural minerals during processing but these minerals are then used to make health supplements. artificial chemical version is normally used in mass produced processed foods to keep the cost of production down.

Natural salt provides the highest nutrition. Salt intake is essential for good health.

Serotonin is a chemical generated in the brain that relays messages around the brain. However as 90% of serotonin is found in the digestive area and blood platelets this suggests food has a big interaction with this chemical. It is widely understood in the medical industry that a lack of serotonin leads to depression and doctors prescribe medicine as a solution.

Serenity describes a peaceful way of thinking about how to handle life there is a serenity verse. "Please grant me the serenity to accept the things I cannot change, the wisdom to know the

difference, Courage to change the things I can."
There are other similar versions of this verse
which became popular through AA (Alcoholics
Anonymous) first teachings in 1930's with a
highly successful 12 step recovery to addiction
program.

Sciatica comes from the sciatic nerves which
run down the legs. When the nerve get slightly
trapped "Trapped Nerve" the pain can be very
acute. It took me around ten years to understand
how to treat sciatica (without an operation) which
had previously ruled my life, dictating when I was
able to walk.

Side effects from medicines are common and
expected especially from the stronger prescribed
ones. The manufacturer publishes the side
effects are printed on the packaging with extra
information enclosed in the packets.

Keeping aware of the side effects is helpful to
know so you have a sense of knowing why your
body is behaving in a certain way.

The medical industry promotes the view point
of do the benefits of the medicine outweigh any
unwanted side effects. Keep asking questions,
learning more about your prescribed medicines
in case you come across better options.

Sleep apnea is a sleeping disorder due to lack
of breathing oxygen the body wakes up. This is

very tiring. High blood is a common associated un-wellness with sleep apnea sufferers. This condition is more likely with obese men.

Spiritual is often mentioned in the common phase "mind body and spirit" for the purpose of this book in step 11. It means anything non physical, it's all encompassing good energy. This does not mean having to be be religious or believing in a God.

Sugar naturally is produced in fruit. The organic fruit is better to consume as it has not been sprayed with pesticides. Pesticides sprayed on fruit makes the plant too toxic for insects to live on. Sugar is present in most plants and is extracted large quantities from sugar cane. As sugar has an addictive nature consumers experience a sugar high followed by a dip or withdrawal which stimulates more consumption.

Sugar High, Fix, Rush describes a boost of energy from consuming sugar usually in a concentrated form such as chocolate, biscuits and sugary deserts. It take about 15 minutes to feel the sugar high. One experiment with mice showed they preferred sugar to cocaine.

Stomach chemicals involved with digesting foods are able to send back signals to the brain about how full the stomach is. This takes about 15 -30 minutes for the stomach to acknowledge it is full to the brain. By eating slower it gives the stomach enough time to let the brain know it is full with a natural speed of digestion.

Stress at high levels causing un-wellness begins when a person is presented with more than their comfortable level of physical, emotional or mental ability to handle life events. Short term your body makes a healthy reaction by producing adrenaline. These repeated bursts of adrenaline during each day start to wears out the glands long term. The adrenaline rush may become normal or addictive.

Long term high stress turns into physical un-wellness so watch out for the warning symptoms of:

- Low energy or a fatigue condition
- Headaches or migraine
- Indigestion , diarrhoea, constipation, nausea
- Tense muscles, aches, pains
- Chest pain and rapid heartbeat
- Insomnia
- Regular colds and infections
- Nervousness tremors, ringing in the ear, cold or sweaty hands and feet
- Dry mouth and difficulty swallowing
- Clenched jaw and grinding teeth day or night

Getting a new approach to chronic stress is essential for restoring a healthy digestive function so the digestive enzymes are maximising the nutrition.

Detoxing sleep, high nutrition and moderate exercise reduce stress so the brain is best able to function. No part of the body is immune from the long term un-wellness from high stress. Taking detoxing holidays may help diagnosis the root cause of un-wellness by having time to physically and mentally relax.

Sugar - white has undergone a bleaching process to take out the brown colour and therefore the original nutrition. White sugar is a popular colour and is the most widely sold.

Sunlight is essential for wellbeing and gives us vitamin D. When someone is not able to go outside for medical reasons or is suffering from a low nutrition lifestyle doctors often prescribe a vitamin D supplement. In winter time when there is less sunlight some people suffer depression from lack of sunlight.

Sweeteners are a sugar substitute made from artificial chemicals.

Taste Buds in the mouth are on the upper surface of the tongue which sense the five tastes which are salty, sour, bitter, sweet and umami.

Tea tree soap is a soap with the essential oil tea tree which is known for natural healing properties on skin.

TENS machine technology Transcutaneous Electrical Nerve Stimulation. This is a small portable machine used for pain relief. It gives out small electrical signals. It boosts circulation. This is an important gadget when exercise is not very possible due to physical disability.

Tinnitus is a health condition that causes the sufferer constant ringing in their ears.

Toxic or Toxicity describes a substance which can damage an organism.

Unami is one of the five tastes human beings experience the other four are sweetness, sourness, bitterness, and saltiness.

Vaccinations are medications to prevent catching diseases by providing immunity. Before having a vaccination it is worth checking any known side effects. Some vaccinations have been banned. These are a very important part of modern day medicine which has saved many lives and often are taken for travelling abroad where different countries have high and low risks of disease such as malaria. When possible it is worth checking how long a drug has been on the market.

Vegetarian and Vegan describes people who consume a vegetable diet there are many variations to this. This lifestyle of diet is on the increase in The U.K.

www.vegansociety.com

Vegetables which are frozen means their nutrition value is locked in.

Vegetables cooked with (99%+) purified water in a sealed pressure cooker lock in the maximum nutrition.

Vitamin B and the different types of B vitamins associated with the well-being of the brain functions are accepted as beneficial backed up by research. For mental well-being from foods and increased happiness levels see Serotonin and **Dopamine**.

Vitamin C is commonly associated with Oranges especially in advertising. This vitamin is very good at healing because it builds the immunity. Taking tablets as a supplement is a very common habit for people on low nutrition diets. It is most important to maximise the way vitamin C is absorbed into the body. It is not possible to overdose on this as the body expels excess.

Vitamin D is gained from sunlight. Lack of it can happen from staying permanently indoors. There are vitamin D supplements which offer a good medical alternative when the person is unable to access sunlight easily. Some skins absorb vitamin D better than others.

Washing Food with tap water means adding several of the artificial chemicals in the water to the food. For example tap water needs weeds killer to ensure the pipes do not get clogged up. There are many chemicals in the water. Usually the water board in the UK, European countries & USA publish facts about the local tap water.

Water Purified means it is 99% free of contaminants.

Water Bottled low priced bottled water sold in shops not stating the source as Spring or Mineral is tap water ! The natural better option is Spring and mineral water. However to purify (99%+) water through your own home system or mobile filters is the cheapest way to be sure of acquire high quality water lowest cost.

Water content in The Human Body is made up of about 60% depending on age and size. The organs in the body such as the liver have a much higher water content partly due to their detoxing, filtering functions.

Water tap has to travel along way through pipes and weeds must not block the pipes so a mild weed killer has to be added to the water supply.

Other chemicals are added at the pumping station to kill bacteria.

Willpower alone is very unlikely to be enough to give up any strong addiction long term. Attempted lifestyle changes based mainly on personal will power usually work only short term. An improved peaceful feeling of serenity has proven to be the best approach for overcoming addictions long term. This has been proven with the high success rate of from the many well known 12 step addiction recovery programs which were first published in 1939.

WONDEA a six level nutrition hierarchy of needs to describe this 80/20 % 12 step chemaholic recovery plan as follows:

- **W**ater   purified
- **O**rganic   vegetables
- **N**atural   products foods, drinks
  and skin
  contact
- **D**etoxification   sleep, skin, air
  treatments
- **E**xercise   movement, circulation
- **A**rtificial chemicals   nutrition and products

World Health Organisation (WHO) was setup 1948 to regulate and help make recommendations to its members which are countries. They are an independent global health organisation.   www.who.int/en/

All the answers to the quiz questions are in this section. How about have some fun making your own Chemaholic quiz so I have added lots more answers to quiz your friends with !

WONDEA

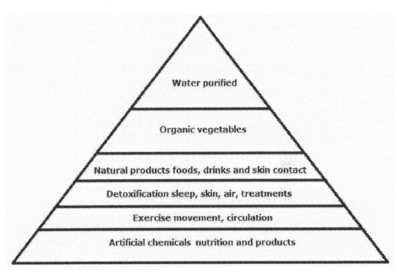

Six level nutrition hierarchy of needs describe this 80% Natural nutrition & 20% artificial nutrition 12 step chemaholic recovery plan as follows:

- **W**ater purified
- **O**rganic vegetables
- **N**atural products foods, drinks and skin contact
- **D**etoxification treatments sleep, skin, air
- **E**xercise movement, circulation
- **A**rtificial chemicals nutrition and products

Benefits of Processed Food Nutrition

(Made with artificial chemicals and pesticides)

- The fast growing world population copes better with processed food production to satisfy demand.

- This kind of food can be found quickly– and requires low or no preparation time.

- Processed food is inexpensive – mass production, bulk distribution, cheap ingredients make products low cost(excluding brand name products which have high marketing costs to build into the product price)

- Products can easily be transported long distances to places where there is no or little food available from natural sources—for example, long boat journeys or places with extreme weather conditions, after natural disasters and wars.

- Processed food is convenient because it is ready-made and packaged in easy-to-consume ways.

- This food is easy to distribute to shops and often has longer shop shelf life.

- The low nutrition food industry employs a lot of people throughout the world and supports many charities often local to the production where otherwise there could be financial hardship.

- The low nutrition industry sponsors many worthwhile events, including sports.

- With world population increasing, bigger supplies of all types of nutrition are required to keep up with demand, especially processed foods and, more recently, synthetic foods.

Dictionary Definitions in Full

Chemicalism

Chemicalism The subject of artificial chemically processed food and drink addictive dependence by human beings and animals.

Full. Characterised when (Chemaholics) with regular compulsive cravings, loss of control over the consumption of artificially chemically processed foods drinks, continue consumption despite negative consequences and withdrawal upon stopping consumption. The Chemaholic continues consumption of addictive chemically processed foods which is both rewarding and reinforcing. Studies have shown this addictive condition applies to animals and human beings. Chemicalism involves the addition of artificially made chemicals at any stage in the process of making a food or drink. History. 1962 The European Union started defining food additives with "E Numbers" which has been adopted by many countries to regulate processed food production and information stated on product packaging. For example, E number E621 defines Monosodium glutamate created in 1908 by Japanese Chemist Professor Ikeda Kikunae. E954 Saccharin the first artificial sweetener synthesized in 1879 by Remsen and Fahlberg. E250 Sodium nitrite is one of many preservatives used to extend shelf life of food and drinks. Wars by land and sea (<u>French Navy 1806</u>) stimulated the necessity to invent methods to preserve food and drinks by canning to sustain soldiers fighting ability over longer geographical distance. Vacuum sealed cans were invented 1873.After WWII, <u>consumerism</u> and globalization of trading stimulated the increase of Chemicalism through mass market factory production, distributing to food shops later supermarkets. The increased success of global marketing through media, branding, attractively enticing, conveniently packaged processed food and drinks brought about rapid growth of Chemicalism. There are many benefits of processed food and drinks using artificial food additives, including lower cost of production, easy distribution, consumer convenience, reduced preparation time and longer shelf life preservation.

Slang. The phrases "processed foods" or "junk foods" are often used loosely as slang to describe food and drink products created with artificial chemicals typically containing high amounts of one, two or three ingredients labelled as sugar/sweetener, fat, and salt. During the Chemicalization process, nutrition values of the original natural products are altered.

Note Opposite. It is possible to create natural processed foods using natural additives including preservatives—for example, natural sea salt. Natural colourings example beetroot. Many natural foods and drinks have been prepared using processes for many hundreds of years such as raw coffee beans (grown without artificial fertiliser or pesticides) which are roasted into a consumable form with no artificial chemicals. For the purpose of defining Chemicalism, processed food and drink products include artificial chemicals.

Chemicalism and the resulting medical condition Chemaholic was defined by British born Simon Kadwill-Kelly in 2013 a self confessed long term Chemaholic who started recovery (under doctors supervision) during six months in 2013 by changing to natural nutrition of mainly organic foods and purified water which lead to significant weight loss, no longer being classified obese, no longer with high cholesterol. This same natural diet was followed by Simon Kadwill-Kelly's mother who became cured of illnesses most significantly being cured of terminal Gangrene of the foot avoiding an amputation of the leg and diabetes type II at 94 years old. Greek. Pronounced "Kemicall ism".

Chemaholic: A person or animal suffering from Chemicalism. Also Chemiholic same meaning. When a Chemaholic has regular compulsive cravings, loss of control over the consumption, continued consumption despite negative consequences and withdrawal upon stopping consumption of processed food and drinks made (chemicalized) with artificial chemicals. The Chemaholic continues consumption regularly or on a regular Binge basis of addictive chemically processed foods which is both rewarding and reinforcing. The person or animal may not be aware they are a Chemaholic. Yale Food Addiction Scale (YFAS) indicates some people have a higher risk to food addiction. Side effects for a suffering Chemaholic. Medical health tests for human beings confirming conditions of high cholesterol, high blood pressure, high sugar levels associated with being or becoming diabetic, circulation illnesses, autoimmunity illness, obesity provide the Chemaholic with their own diagnosis of evidence of illness suffering. The retesting typically with blood testing after a withdrawal of several weeks from a Chemaholic Lifestyle indicates the diagnosis and solution. This was defined by British born Simon Kadwill-Kelly in 2013 a self confessed long term Chemaholic. He mainly recovered from un wellness and obesity in six months (recorded in medical notes) during 2013 by changing to natural nutrition of mainly organic foods and purified water as guided by Elsa Wakeling who had followed a lifestyle of Naturopathy. This same diet was followed by Simon Kadwill-Kelly's mother who then became cured of illnesses including terminal Gangrene of the foot. Greek. Pronounced "Kemaholic" or "Kemiholic".

References

1. E Numbers. Cambridge English Dictionary. Any of a set of numbers with the letter E in front of them that are used on containers of food in the European Union to show which particular approved chemical has been added to the food. http://dictionary.cambridge.org/

2. E Number definitions for each one.UK Food Standards Agency FSA List. https://www.food.gov.uk/science/additives/enumberlist

3. Addiction. September 2014.Joseph Schroeder, Associate Professor of Psychology and Director of the Behavioural Neuroscience Program, Connecticut College, led Honohan and other students in the experiment, which led to the conclusion that rats find Oreos Cookies just as addictive as cocaine.

http://www.washingtonpost.com/blogs/answer-sheet/wp/2013/10/18/rats-find-oreos-as-addictive-as-cocaine-an-unusual-college-research-project/

4. Marketing. September 2014.The World Health Organisation (WHO) Protecting children from the harmful effects of food and drink marketing.

http://www.who.int/features/2014/uk-food-drink-marketing/en/

5. Addiction. 2010 study conducted by scientists at Scripps Research Institute (SRI) in Florida found that rats given free access to artificial processed foods had brain activity and function mirroring those occurring in the brains of drug addicts.

http://www.scripps.edu/news/
press/2010/20100329.html

6. Addiction. Sugar. Neurobiology research shows food causes serious addiction, the kind that addictive drugs do. Dr Nicole Avena and colleagues, the Department of Psychiatry, University of Florida, report the consumption of sugar not only alters brain function and behaviour; it also elicits the same type of withdrawal symptoms like opiate drugs do. Sugar affects the opioid receptors in the brain, which are recognized by natural (endogenous or not) opioid substances. Foods rich in fat affect the brain in a different way; they cause withdrawal-type symptoms as well. Studies show there is a unique relationship between emotional balance and fatty acids.

7. Addiction. Psychological "High".2011. Researchers at both the University of Texas in Austin (UT) and the Oregon Research Institute found prolonged consumption of junk foods results in reduced activity in the striatum, a section of the forebrain that registers reward the same as with illicit drugs, those addicted to junk food require ever-increasing amounts to get the same "high."

http://www.naturalnews.com/034478_junk_foods_addictive_brain_chemistry.html

8. Addiction. Fat. Study published in The Journal of Clinical Investigation in 2011 tested the effects of fat consumption in healthy people while experiencing experimentally induced sad feelings. Within minutes the sad feelings were significantly alleviated and the subjects reported improved mood, while MRI scans confirmed the expected brain response. This study is important as it shows fat does not have to be properly digested to modify brain functions. The presence of fat in the gut triggers the release of gastrointestinal hormones, which regulate neurological and emotional responses within minutes.

http://www.jci.org/articles/view/46380

9. Addiction. Brain Dopamine Levels and Obesity. Study 2001 Gene-Jack Wang and Nora Volkow of the Brookhaven National Laboratory.

http://www.thelancet.com/journals/lancet/article/PIIS0140-6736(00)03643-6/abstract

10. World Health Organisation (WHO) Global Strategy on Diet, Physical Activity and Health" was adopted in 2004 by the World Health Assembly (WHA). It called on governments, WHO, international partners, the private sector and civil society to take action at global, regional and local levels to support healthy diets and physical activity.

http://www.who.int/mediacentre/factsheets/fs394/en/

11. Yale Food Addiction Scale (YFAS) is a 25-point questionnaire, based on DSM-IV codes for substance dependence criteria, to assess food addiction in individuals. The scale was released in 2009 by Yale University's Rudd Centre for Food Policy and Obesity.

12. www.Chemicalism.org an ongoing long term growing reference.

Books and Websites

Cut the Crap and Feel Amazing (2014)
how to let go of the negative and get into the amazing zone
Ailsa Frank

Love Life – Eat Well
Riki-Davies

The Gut
Jane Plant's Testimonial preventing and treating cancer

You Can Heal Your Life
Louise L. Hay

Easy Way To Stop Smoking
Allen Carr

Feel the Fear and Do It Anyway
Susan Jeffers

Health Nutrition Secrets
Russell L Blaylock M.D. Neurosurgeon

To find a reliable list of useful books, DVDs, CDs, and publications in different formats plus free information with regular free updates, visit:

NHS Blood donation
www.blood.co.uk

Cancer Research
www.cancerresearchuk.org

Chemicalism since 2013
www.chemicalism.org

Chemaholic since 2013
www.chemaholic.org

Detoxing products on sale
www.detoxlifestyle.co.uk

General Naturopathic Council
www.gncouncil.co.uk

The Vegan Society
www.vegansociety.com

The World Health Organisation
www.who.int

Medical Notes

The weight measurements held in my NHS medical notes show I lost around 18 kilos in six month, three years ago. This has remained about the same.

I started my preparation with exercising a lot January - March 2013 with no new knowledge about food. This was hard work, involving some food deprivation but I managed to lose around 4 kilos. Then I went to Morocco for a holiday and quickly put weight on again. I was ready for something new.

| | | Blood Pressure | | BMI | Weight | |
		Systolic	Diastolic		Kilo	Stone Pounds
Get Active programme 12 weeks (pre)	22/04/2013	136	90	34.71	102.7	17.47
Get Active programme 12 weeks later	15/07/2013	110	92	32.04	94.8	16.77
Medical Notes	20/01/2014	X	X	28.8	86	13.54
Medical Notes	24/10/2014	X	X	27.9	85.5	13.46
Nurse	22/05/2016	110	65	27.8	85.4	13.44

I started the Get Active referral programme 22/4/2013 after my doctor gave me a free NHS prescription to exercise! The exercise sessions were at my local leisure centre with Magda my personal trainer. We also talked about natural foods and how I could incorporate them into a new lifestyle.

At the end of the 12 week programme my weight and blood pressure were rechecked. My blood pressure had gone down with no medication.

The Get Active programme is funded by Sport England who distributes around £300 million pounds every year. Sport England receives about one quarter of funding from the U.K. government with the balance from The National Lottery. They aim to increase the number of people doing sport and activity whatever someone's background, ability or age.

Measuring your blood pressure, glucose and body weight at home can be done with good equipment. Most people have a pair of scales but it is good to check they are accurate.

Summary

This is the book I wanted to buy in 2013 whilst desperately searching for the natural solutions to:

- Easily overcome my obesity long term
- Find a natural cure for terminal gangrene and diabetes for my mum

There wasn't anything simple available in 2013 that took a non technical approach and covered having a new attitude in the same book. I could find excellent cook books easily. Also there were many long in depth psychology books by medical experts but I was in a hurry.

This is a simple positive easy to follow Lifestyle 12 step plan based around enjoying tasty high and low nutrition foods with purified water. Balanced with modern day western world living an awareness of chemicals put into people's lifestyles can be easily complimented with everyday detoxing.

No special equipment is required to get started today (except a water purifier investment to save money.)

With a high nutrition lifestyle automatically the body performs better and settles at a natural weight.

An open mind is essential for step one and the other steps falling into place at your own pace.

Everyone has their own preferences for food. It is important to adjust to a high natural nutrition appetite with your own taste buds, satisfied with increased flavour sensitivity.

If you feel step one "*I am crazy*" repeating the same actions everyday expecting a different result is not for you. Then there are thousands of short term calorie controlling and exercise based dieting plans on offer. My suggestion is eat natural foods when possible and drink more purified water.

I believe today's healthy lifestyle balancing trick is to consume high levels of natural nutrition for stronger immunity to:

- Avoid major un wellness
- Strengthen natural detoxing
- Benefit from only minimal medicinal drugs and supplements
- Enjoy favourite convenient choices of food and drink without feeling deprived
- Improve immunity
- Keep shopping and health costs down
- Maximise energy levels

Keep in contact for updates by registering free or ordering any products mentioned.

This book is mainly based on testimonial by myself and my mum. To make this recovery plan more widely acknowledged it needs several thousand people to take part in a study.

Get involved register at www.chemicalism.org or www.chemicalism.com

"It's my good fortune to share the hope and faith I've been shown so far on my journey from obesity to now enjoying a healthier lifestyle. This includes my easy 12 step long term weight loss method that has worked for me. Wishing anything self helpful in this quick read book is easily passed on. It's just about an increased awareness of Chemicalism"

2013

Learning about Chemicalism By enjoying tasty food

13.5stone

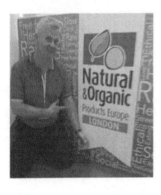

2012

Eating a healthy "looking" salad with tap water in a restaurant

17.5stone

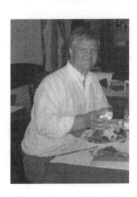

8316121R00169

Printed in Germany
by Amazon Distribution
GmbH, Leipzig